THE ULTIMATE GUIDE AND REVIEW FOR USMLE STEP 2 CLINICAL SKILLS EXAM

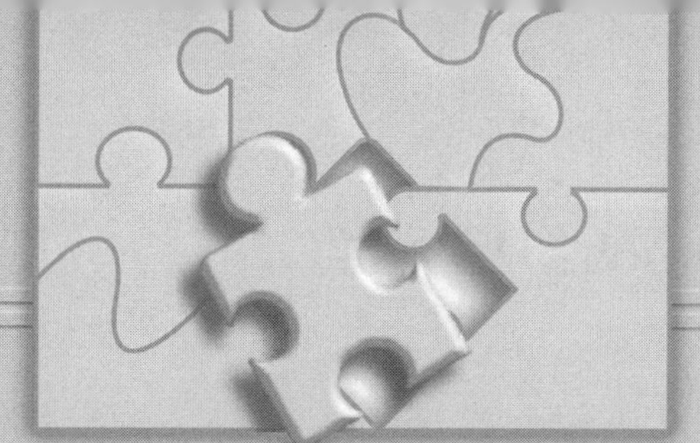

THE ULTIMATE GUIDE AND REVIEW FOR USMLE STEP 2 CLINICAL SKILLS EXAM

Mark H. Swartz, M.D. F.A.C.P.
Professor of Medicine
State University of New York (SUNY)
Downstate College of Medicine
Brooklyn, New York

Founder and Director
C3NY
Clinical Competence Center of New York
New York, New York

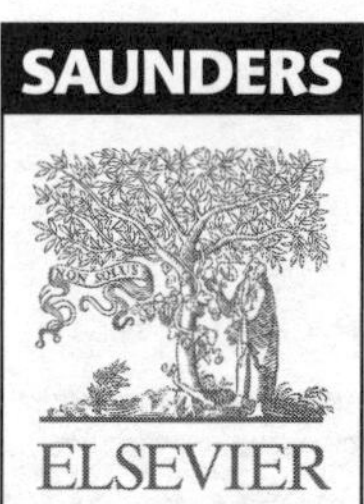

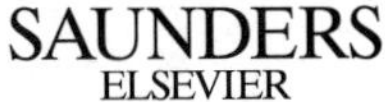

1600 John F. Kennedy Blvd.
Ste 1800
Philadelphia, PA 19103-2899

The Ultimate Guide and Review for the USMLE Step 2 Clinical Skills Exam

ISBN-13: 978-1-4160-3727-9
ISBN-10: 1-4160-3727-6

Notice

Knowledge and best practice in this field are constantly changing. As new research and experience broaden our knowledge, changes in practice, treatment and drug therapy may become necessary or appropriate. Readers are advised to check the most current information provided (i) on procedures featured or (ii) by the manufacturer of each product to be administered, to verify the recommended dose or formula, the method and duration of administration, and contraindications. It is the responsibility of the practitioner, relying on their own experience and knowledge of the patient, to make diagnoses, to determine dosages and the best treatment for each individual patient, and to take all appropriate safety precautions. To the fullest extent of the law, neither the Publisher nor the Author assumes any liability for any injury and/or damage to persons or property arising from or related to any use of the material contained in this book.

The Publisher

Library of Congress Cataloging-in-Publication Data

Swartz, Mark H.

The ultimate guide and review for USMLE step 2 clinical skills exam / Mark H. Swartz

p. cm.

ISBN 1-4160-3727-6

1. Diagnosis—Examinations, questions, etc. 2. Medical history taking—Examinations, questions, etc. 3. Physical diagnosis—Examinations, questions, etc. 4. Physicians—Licenses—United States—Examinations—Study guides. I. Title.

RC71.S93 2007

616.07'5076—dc22

2006047588

Acquisitions Editor: William Schmitt
Editorial Assistant: Kevin Kochanski
Publishing Services Manager: Linda Van Pelt
Project Manager: Melanie Peirson Johnstone
Design Direction: Ellen Zanolle

Printed in United States of America

Last digit is the print number: 9 8 7 6 5 4 3 2 1

To **Vivian Hirshaut, MD**,
my wife, my life's companion and my best friend,
for her love, support, and understanding;

To **Talia H. Swartz, PhD**,
my wonderful and devoted daughter,
who is pursuing her studies toward her MD degree;

To the memory of my parents,
Hilda and **Philip Swartz**;

and

To my **students**,
from whom I am always learning.

Preface

It took me several years to decide to write this book. Because of my extensive experience with standardized patients, about 5 years ago I was approached by a few publishers to write a book to prepare candidates to take the Step 2 Clinical Skills exam. I was undecided; I did not want to produce a book that would merely provide lists of questions to be asked and answers to be given. Good communication is a dynamic skill, requiring careful listening skills that necessitate taking leads from the other person's verbal and nonverbal cues; it can never be planned! All conversation needs to ebb and flow between the interviewer and the patient.

I finally realized that the demand for this text outweighed my hesitation. So I resolved to produce a guidebook that incorporates my firmly held beliefs, supported by the passing outcomes of my many students, that this exam is first and foremost an assessment of communication skills, and that it cannot be approached by sheer memorization.

Taking high-stakes examinations in general are anxiety-provoking experiences. The USMLE Step 2 Clinical Skills exam is unlike any other test you have ever taken, and it is frequently the source of much stress. This practical exam assesses your proficiency in history taking, physical examination, and communication/interpersonal skills through the use of standardized patients.

The ***Ultimate Guide and Review for USMLE Step 2 Clinical Skills Exam*** will guide you through all aspects of this new-format examination. In addition to informing you about the important concepts of the exam, it suggests many of the communication techniques that are so vital in establishing an excellent doctor–patient relationship. A brief cultural guide will provide some information about the American culture—the laws, practices, and etiquette—to avoid potentially embarrassing and costly miscues when dealing with the American patient. The 30 practice cases will help you hone your history-taking, physical examination, and communication skills, and help you develop the confidence needed to be successful on the examination. Being well prepared makes the exam a less stressful experience.

Although I have provided you with 30 practice cases, I have not listed a "how to" in your approach to these cases (i.e., questions and responses). **Step 2 Clinical Skills is an exam about communication skills**; I cannot emphasize this enough! Each interaction is distinctive and unpredictable; it needs to be a real conversation, so I think it ill advised to memorize questions and responses.

Since 1990, I have had an ongoing relationship with members of the National Board of Medical Examiners (NBME) as well as with the Educational Commission for Foreign Medical Graduates (ECFMG). My medical education research in standardized patient assessment contributed to the development of the national licensing exams. I would like you to understand, however, that the information provided in this book is from my experience as an educator and does not reflect any direct connection between these organizations and this book.

Over the past 16 years, I have prepared more than 20,000 medical students and international medical graduates to take standardized patient examinations, and I continue to do so. I understand what is needed for success on these assessments; I am delighted to share my knowledge with you.

I wish you good luck on your exam.

Mark H. Swartz, MD

Acknowledgments

I wish to thank all my American medical students and international medical graduates who have helped in providing suggestions for this book.

I would like to thank the many employees of Elsevier for their expert assistance. In particular, I wish to acknowledge William Schmitt, my editor/publishing director, and the production team of Melanie Peirson Johnstone and Ellen Zanolle.

I want to thank Margaret Clark Golden, MD, Associate Professor of Pediatrics at the State University of New York (SUNY) Downstate College of Medicine, for helping in the development of the pediatric case.

I owe a debt of gratitude to Anna Lank, the Assistant Director of C3NY, the Clinical Competence Center of New York, for her tireless support, enthusiasm, and assistance in helping with the development of all the cases in this book and in providing suggestions for the text. This book has been enhanced greatly by her contributions and guidance.

Finally, I want to thank my wife, Vivian Hirshaut, MD, and my daughter, Talia H. Swartz, PhD, for their constant support and encouragement, which made this book a reality.

Mark H. Swartz, MD

About the Author

Mark H. Swartz, MD, is recognized nationally and internationally for his teaching ability and has received many teaching awards. He has been working in the medical area of clinical simulation with standardized patients for over 15 years, and his work in this field laid the groundwork for the current national licensing board examination. His research over the past 15 years has centered on improving medical education and assessment of clinical competence. He has published more than 50 seminal articles in this area, and is one of the world's leading authorities on standardized patient assessment.

Dr. Swartz was graduated from New York University and received his medical degree from Mount Sinai School of Medicine, where he was selected for Alpha Omega Alpha. He is currently Professor of Medicine at the State University of New York (SUNY) Downstate College of Medicine. Previously, he spent more than three decades at the Mount Sinai School of Medicine, where he was the first Marietta and Charles C. Morchand Professor of Medical Education, Professor of Medicine, and Founder and Director of The Morchand Center for Clinical Competence for more than 13 years. During that time, he also founded and directed the New York City Consortium on Clinical Competence.

Dr. Swartz is the author of five textbooks. The fourth edition of his ***Textbook of Physical Diagnosis: History and Examination*** (now in its fifth edition) was reviewed for the second time in the *New England Journal of Medicine* (July 10, 2003), which cited this new edition as "the most accurate, up-to-date, and comprehensive textbook of physical diagnosis available today." It is the most widely read textbook in this field, and has been translated into six foreign languages.

Since 1990, Dr. Swartz's successful standardized patient programs have educated more than 20,000 American-trained medical students and internationally trained medical graduates. Since the inception of the national licensing examination for international medical graduates in 1998, he has traveled throughout North America teaching doctors how to prepare for these exams with his clinical skills workshops.

In 2004, Dr. Swartz founded C3NY, the Clinical Competence Center of New York (www.c3ny.org). This educational service organization, headquartered in New York City, provides monthly programs to prepare international medical graduates and American-trained medical students to take the USMLE Step 2 Clinical Skills examination. In addition, C3NY provides area medical schools a variety of curricula geared to improve excellence in clinical competence.

Contents

Section 3

Section 4

Section 1

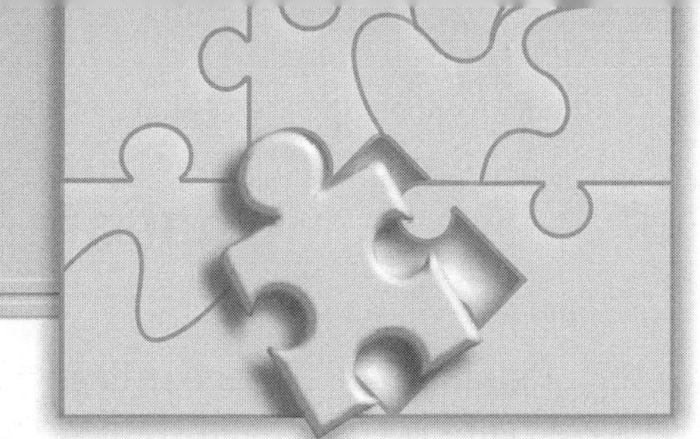

The Basics About the USMLE Step 2 CS Examination

Background Information

The **United States Medical Licensing Examination** (USMLE[1]) is a three-step assessment of a candidate's clinical knowledge and clinical skills and is required for medical licensure in the United States. It is sponsored by the Federation of State Medical Boards (FSMB) and the National Board of Medical Examiners (NBME). *Step 1* assesses whether the candidate understands and can apply important concepts of the basic sciences to the practice of medicine. *Step 2* assesses whether the candidate can apply medical knowledge, skills, and understanding of clinical science essential for provision of patient care under supervision. *Step 3* assesses whether the candidate can apply medical knowledge and understanding of biomedical and clinical science essential for the unsupervised practice of medicine.

Step 2 consists of two separate examinations: *Step 2 CK* (Clinical Knowledge) and *Step 2 CS* (Clinical Skills). *Step 2 CK* consists of multiple choice questions to determine the candidate's clinical knowledge deemed essential for the provision of patient care under supervision in postgraduate training. *Step 2 CS* is a practical examination using *standardized patients* to test a candidate's proficiency to gather information from patients, perform physical examinations, and communicate effectively with patients and colleagues.

The results of the three Steps of the USMLE are reported to the medical licensing authorities in the United States for the purpose of granting or denying initial medical licensure.

---

[1]USMLE is a joint program of the Federation of State Medical Boards of the United States, Inc. and the National Board of Medical Examiners.

What are Standardized Patients?

The standardized patients do not evaluate your medical knowledge; they merely record that which transpired during the clinical encounter.

Standardized patients, or ***SPs***, are individuals (often actors) who have been trained to simulate the signs and symptoms of disease and trained to give feedback and/or accurately record the details of an interaction. They are selected from a wide range of ages and racial and ethnic backgrounds. The SPs do *not* evaluate your medical knowledge; they merely record that which transpired during a clinical encounter. You are expected to treat the SP as a real patient while demonstrating excellent communication skills in an empathic and professional manner.

For the past 10 years, most medical schools in the United States and Canada that are accredited by the Liaison Committee on Medical Education (LCME) have used standardized patients for instruction; many of these institutions use standardized patients for evaluation as well. Since July 1998, standardized patients have been used in the Educational Commission for Foreign Medical Graduates (ECFMG) Certification process with their Clinical Skills Assessment (CSA). Step 2 CS replaced the CSA formerly administered by the ECFMG. Effective June 14, 2004, Step 2 CS is a requirement for ECFMG Certification of international medical graduates who have not passed the CSA as well as for all individuals wishing to practice medicine in the United States.

The standardized patients used on the national licensing examinations undergo rigorous training.

SPs have also been incorporated into the Medical Council of Canada's medical licensure examination for Canadian and international medical graduates for many years. The use of SPs as a standardized assessment method was established more than 30 years ago, and their use in medical education and assessment has been tested and validated in the United States and internationally. The SPs used on the national licensing examinations undergo rigorous training, and although you need to treat them as if they are real patients, they are professionals and are trained as experienced evaluators.

The use of well-trained and reliable SPs ensures that all examinees receive the same information when they ask the patients the same or similar questions. An ongoing mechanism of quality control is employed to ensure that the examination is fair to all candidates.

The purpose of the USMLE Step 2 CS Examination is to test your proficiency on your clinical skills of history taking, physical examination, and communication—not in making a diagnosis! It evaluates your ability to gather data from your patients. Unlike other written or

Purpose of Step 2 CS

Examination Length

The exam is approximately 8 hours in length with two breaks. The first break is 30 minutes long, and the second is 15 minutes long. Each day, there is a morning and afternoon session, and there may be two simultaneous sessions in the morning and in the afternoon. Candidates are organized into groups of 11 or 12 and rotate through the 11 or 12 cases.

You may use the restroom before the exam and during breaks. A light meal is provided during the first break, and there are vending machines available for drinks. Vegetarian food is available. You can bring your own food, provided that no refrigeration or preparation is required. Smoking is prohibited throughout the center.

computer examinations, it is a practical examination using standardized patients and measures different skill sets than traditional multiple-choice examinations.

Examination Format

There are 11 or 12 patient encounters, with 11 encounters being scored. The twelfth case is for pilot testing a new case (for validation) or for research purposes. This pilot case is not counted toward your score. This nonscored encounter could be your first, your last, or somewhere in the middle. Each patient encounter is 15 minutes in length and is followed by the writing of a Patient Note. You are allowed 10 minutes to write the note, either on a computer or by hand. Even if you plan to use a computer, make sure that your handwriting is legible in case the computer becomes unavailable as a result of technical or administrative problems.

Each of the 11 or 12 patient encounters is 15 minutes in length and is followed by the writing of a Patient Note. You are allowed 10 minutes to write the note either by hand or on a computer.

The cases represent relatively common presentation categories including, but not limited to, cardiovascular, respiratory, digestive, genitourinary, neurologic, psychiatric, constitutional, and other areas (e.g., ear, eyes, nose, throat, musculoskeletal, women's health, men's health). Examinees will see cases from some, but not all, of these categories. On any specific examination day, the set of cases differs from the combination presented the day before or the following day, but each set of cases has a comparable degree of difficulty.

Legibility counts!

Eligibility for Step 2 CS

To be eligible, you must be in one of the following categories at the time of application and on the test day:

- a medical student officially enrolled in, or a graduate of, a U.S. or Canadian medical school program leading to the MD degree that is accredited by the LCME;
- a medical student officially enrolled in, or a graduate of, a U.S. medical school program leading to the DO degree that is accredited by the American Osteopathic Association (AOA); or
- a medical student officially enrolled in, or a graduate of, a medical school outside the United States and Canada and eligible for examination by the ECFMG for its certificate.

Once eligibility requirements are met, you may take Step 1, Step 2 CK, and Step 2 CS in any sequence.

Step 2 CS is offered regularly throughout the year. There is no deadline for submitting your application to register for Step 2 CS. Be aware, however, that demand for test dates/centers at certain times during the year may exceed the number of testing spaces available.

Step 2 CS Registration

Registration information is frequently modified. For the most current registration information, go to www.usmle.org. Registration for students and graduates of medical schools in the United States and Canada is through the **NBME:**

3750 Market Street
Philadelphia, PA 19104-3190
Telephone: (215) 590-9700
Fax: (215) 590-9457 FAX
Web Address: http://www.nbme.org
Email: webmail@nbme.org

Registration for students and graduates of medical schools outside the USA and Canada is through the **ECFMG:**

3624 Market Street
Philadelphia, PA 19104-2685
Telephone: (215) 386-5900
Fax: (215) 386-9196
Web Address: http://www.ecfmg.org
Email: info@ecfmg.org

Applicants registered for Step 2 CS are assigned a 12-month eligibility period that begins when the processing of their application is completed. This eligibility period is listed on your **Step 2 CS Scheduling Permit,** which you will receive by e-mail after the application is processed. The Scheduling Permit contains the following information:

- your name and mailing address;
- your USMLE identification number;
- your eligibility period;
- instructions for scheduling your testing appointment;
- a description of the identification required for admission to the testing center.

You must take the exam during your eligibility period. You can schedule a testing appointment for any available date or location during your eligibility period. Once your eligibility period is assigned, it cannot be changed. If you do *not* take the exam within your eligibility period, you must reapply to take the exam, including repayment of the examination fee. Although you cannot change your assigned eligibility period, you can reschedule a scheduled testing appointment within your eligibility period.

In addition to your Scheduling Permit, you will receive a CD-ROM that contains an orientation manual and video presentations of sample SP encounters.

To receive ECFMG certification, **international medical graduates** need to pass Step 1, Step 2 CK, and Step 2 CS within a 7-year period. For the purpose of ECFMG Certification, there is no limit on the number of times you can take a Step or Step Component you have not passed. You must be certified by ECFMG if you wish to take Step 3 of the three-step USMLE.

Fees for Step 2 CS

The examination fee for medical students in the United States and Canada is currently US$975; the fee for international graduates is currently US$1,200. Fees, including cancellation and rescheduling fees, are subject to change. Check the USMLE web site for current information about fees.

Location of Regional Clinical Skills Evaluation Centers

There are five regional Clinical Skills Evaluation Centers. You can select the center where you will take the exam. The centers are currently located in Philadelphia, Atlanta, Houston, Los Angeles, and Chicago.

Philadelphia
3624 Market Street
Philadelphia, PA 19104

Atlanta
Two Crown Center
1745 Phoenix Boulevard
Suite 500
Atlanta, GA 30349

Houston
400 North Belt
400 North Sam Houston Parkway
Suite 700
Houston, TX 77060

Los Angeles
Pacific Corporate Towers
13th Floor
100 North Sepulveda Boulevard
El Segundo, CA 90245

Chicago
Crossroads Center at O'Hare
6th Floor
8501 West Higgins Road
Chicago, IL 60018

Selecting Exam Time and Place

You should register and schedule your exam as soon as possible. Testing spaces are filled on a "first-come, first served" basis.

You should register and schedule your exam as soon as possible. The examination is administered in both morning and afternoon sessions. You are able to select a date and center, but not the test session. You will be assigned to either the morning or afternoon session. Once the morning slots fill up, they begin to fill the afternoon ones. Testing spaces are filled on a "first-come, first served" basis. The spaces in the centers may be allocated based on a variety of factors, including time of year, location of the test center, and whether the examinee's institution of undergraduate medical education is located within the United States, Canada, or is an international medical school. Controls on the spaces for each test session remain in place until 60 days before the test date, at which time all testing spaces that have not been filled are made available to all registered applicants. Scheduling patterns and demand are constantly monitored, and allotment of spaces may be modified at any time.

Rescheduling Exam Dates

Effective June 24, 2005, but subject to change, the following rules govern rescheduling exam dates:

- If you cancel more than 14 calendar days before (but not including) your scheduled test date, there is no fee to reschedule.
- If you cancel during the 14-day period before (but not including) your scheduled test date, your fee will be US$150 when you reschedule.
- If you miss your scheduled testing appointment without canceling, your fee will be US$400 when you reschedule.

Check www.usmle.org for current information regarding rescheduling exam dates.

Scoring of Step 2 CS

The SP completes checklists that document your skills in history taking, physical examination, and communication.

After each encounter, the SP completes *checklists* that document your skills in history taking, physical examination, and communication. In addition, the SP uses rating scales to assess your English-speaking skills. The Patient Note is read by a physician who evaluates the quality of the documentation, as well as the differential diagnosis and management plans. The physician reads the Patient Note without knowledge of how the candidate performed with the SP (i.e., the checklists). The physician is looking for a clear description of the case: why did the patient come for evaluation, what are the pertinent positives and negatives of the history and physical examination, what is your differential diagnosis, and what are your management plans.

Unlike the other parts of the USMLE that have numerical scores, the score for Step 2 CS is reported as only a PASS or a FAIL.

All interactions are videotaped. The videos of the encounters, however, are *not* reviewed. Videos are used for general quality control and for SP training purposes; they are retained only for a limited period of time. Your score is *never* based on anyone's evaluation of videos from your encounters!

Reporting of Results

New reporting schedule

The results of Step 2 CS are reported by regular mail. In January 2006, a new reporting schedule was established. This schedule calls for results to be reported during specific periods throughout the year, rather than on a rolling basis as done previously. The reporting periods and their corresponding exam dates are found on the USMLE web site (www.usmle.org).

This schedule both enables USMLE staff to improve the score reporting system by enhancing the quality assurance, and provides examinees with guidelines regarding when a result will be reported for a given exam date. These guidelines enable examinees to plan their exam date in order to have their results in time to meet specific deadlines, such as school graduation or "the Match."

There are also periods of the year during which the examination undergoes recalibration. During these periods, the results may take longer to be returned to you.

Score Reporting

The Score Report contains three main areas: Integrated Clinical Encounter (ICE), Communication/Interpersonal Skills (CIS), and Spoken English Proficiency (SEP).

The Score Report contains the following three main areas:

- ***Integrated Clinical Encounter (ICE)*** includes data gathering (history-taking and physical examination checklists) as well as the data sharing (Patient Note). The case-specific checklists are developed by groups of physicians and medical educators. These checklists comprise the essential history and physical examination elements for the specific clinical encounters and are filled out by the SP who has been rigorously trained to do so. All cases are constantly monitored for quality control. The Patient Note is scored by trained physician raters. The note is evaluated for its organization, quality of information, interpretation of data, and legibility.

- ***Communication/Interpersonal Skills (CIS)*** includes the communication checklist. This checklist contains items related to skills in interviewing and collecting information, skills in counseling and delivering information, and your professional manner and your rapport. It is filled out by the SP.
- ***Spoken English Proficiency (SEP)*** includes the spoken English rating scale. This is an evaluation by the SP of the clarity of the candidate's spoken English. Key elements include:
  - Pronunciation
  - Stress, rhythm, and intonation
  - Grammar (especially verb tenses)
  - Repair strategies (Are you able to correct something that was not clear to the patient? You should anticipate that the SP will say that they do not understand you; you should go back and clarify—or *repair*—the question or statement.)
  - Range of vocabulary and sentence structure (Keep it simple!)
  - Listening comprehension errors (Did *you* misunderstand something the patient said?)
  - Listener effort (How difficult is it to understand *you*?)

To receive a passing score on the examination, the candidate must pass all three of the above in a single test administration.

What if I Don't Pass?

You can retake the exam after a minimum of 60 days after the previous test date; however, the exam cannot be taken more than three times within a 12-month period. A new application together with the appropriate fee is required. If for any reason you feel that you have incorrectly received a failing score, you can appeal and request rescoring of the examination. It is, however, unlikely that the ultimate result will change.

On Your Exam Day

Dress conservatively; use deodorant; keep fingernails short

- Dress conservatively and wear comfortable, professional clothing. Men should wear a dress shirt and a tie with long pants.

Women should wear either a dress, blouse and skirt, or a blouse/shirt and slacks. Wear dress shoes; no open-toed shoes or sandals. Western dress is preferable. Do *not* wear clothes that you might commonly wear for a written or computer-based examination. No jeans! Dress professionally!

- Use little perfume or aftershave; use deodorant.
- Wear as little jewelry as possible. Do not wear long earrings.
- If you have long hair, pull it back away from your face.
- Keep your fingernails short.
- Do not chew gum.
- Arrive about 30 minutes before the scheduled time.
- Bring your **Scheduling Permit**, which you will receive when your registration is completed.
- Bring an **unexpired government-issued identification** that includes a photograph and a signature such as a passport, a current driver's license, a national identity card, or an ECFMG-issued identification card. *Your name as it appears on your Scheduling Permit must match the name written in English language characters on your form of identification exactly*. If your identification does not match exactly, you will not be allowed to take the examination.

Bring your Scheduling Permit, unexpired government-issued ID (with photo and signature), clean lab coat, and stethoscope.

- Bring a **clean white laboratory or clinic coat**. If your coat bears your name or the name of a medical institution, the proctors will cover that information with adhesive tape, which you can remove at the end of the testing day.
- Bring your **stethoscope**.
- If you forget to bring a lab coat or stethoscope, it will be provided. However, there are a limited number of these items at each test center. Bring your own; don't risk not having a lab coat or stethoscope.
- No electronic or photographic devices are allowed while taking the examination, including during the breaks. These devices include, but are not limited to, cellular telephones, paging devices, digital watches, two-way communication devices, recording or filming devices, and personal digital assistants (PDAs) such as a Palm Pilot. If you are found to have any of these devices, serious consequences may ensue, and you may jeopardize your licensure. Be sure to leave these items at home because you will not be provided with a secure storage place for them.
- You must follow all of the test center staff's instructions throughout the examination. The examination is monitored through the use of audio and video monitoring and the test proctors. *Failure to follow instructions may result in a determination of irregular behavior and in being barred from taking the USMLE in the future.*
- You will be given a small storage cubicle in which you must place all personal belongings. These cubicles are not secure, so do not bring valuables. Leave any luggage in your hotel and pick it up after the examination.

- There are *no* waiting facilities for family and friends at the center.
- Please be aware that before you begin your exam, you will be asked to sign a Confidentiality Statement regarding the details of the exam.

Each session begins with an orientation. Make sure that you arrive on time. If you arrive during the orientation, you may be allowed to test; however, you will be required to sign a Late Admission Form. If you arrive after the orientation has been completed, you will not be allowed to test. You will have to reschedule your assessment, and you will be required to pay a Rescheduling Fee. Once the orientation has begun, you may not leave the test area until the examination is over.

Your Orientation Session may include a video presentation describing the test center as well as actually showing you an examination room. All questions will be answered by the exam staff.

Follow the proctors' instructions at all times.

Throughout the examination day, staff members/proctors, wearing identifying name tags, will direct you through the examination. You must follow their instructions at all times. You will find that they are very nice and helpful.

Description of the Examination Center

The Clinical Skills Center is similar to a large medical clinic. There is a wide center hall with rooms lining each side, similar to a hall in a hotel. There are 24 examination rooms, 12 on each side. Each room has an examination table, a stool, a wall-mounted oto-ophthalmoscope, a sink, a paper towel dispenser, a trash can, a wall-mounted sphygmomanometer, a wall-mounted Snellen eye chart for 10 feet, a reflex hammer, a tuning fork, a clock, and all the disposable items you might need, including nonlatex gloves. There is a light switch near the ophthalmoscope that will dim the room lights when using the ophthalmoscope. There are also closed circuit securitylike cameras in each of the rooms. All encounters are recorded for the purpose of training and monitoring SP performance. Outside each examination room is a cubicle equipped with a computer, where you will write your Patient Note.

Next to the door, there is a panel that when opened reveals the ***Examinee Instructions***, which includes the basic introductory information about the patient, including the patient's name, age, gender, vital signs, and the reason for visiting the doctor. The vital signs include the blood pressure, which is not necessary to retake unless the patient is hemodynamically or potentially hemodynamically unstable. *Be aware that the reason for seeking medical attention that is provided, however, may* not *be the real reason the patient is coming for medical attention!* Isn't that true in real patient encounters? A patient may tell a triage nurse something, but that is not the real reason for seeking medical consultation. **Be curious**, which is an important attribute of a good physician. There is a copy of the Examinee Instructions in each room.

The center will provide pens and a clipboard with colored paper should you wish to take notes. You may also wish to jot down some notes before you enter the room.

Be aware that the reason for seeking medical attention that is provided on the Examinee Instructions may not be the real reason the patient is coming for medical attention!

Other Important Information about the Exam

- Speak only in English in the test center. Speaking in any other language while in the center is strictly forbidden and will jeopardize your licensure. Proctors monitor all examinee activity.
- Do not discuss the cases with your fellow examinees at any time!
- For each encounter, there will be an announcement 5 minutes before the end of each SP interaction.
- Once you leave the room, you cannot go back in, **SO DON'T LEAVE EARLY!**
- No breast, pelvic, rectal, male genitourinary (GU), or corneal reflex examinations can be performed on the SPs. If these examinations are necessary, include them in the proposed management section in the Patient Note.
- You will be asked to sign a document confirming your willingness to abide with the policies of the USMLE including confidentiality about the examination.
- It is imperative that you follow instructions of the test center proctors throughout the examination. Failure to do so may result in a determination of irregular behavior. The USMLE *Bulletin of Information* provides a complete description of irregular behavior.
- *Do not believe anything you have heard about the content of the cases from anyone!* Take the examination with an open mind.

Once you leave the room, you cannot go back—DON'T LEAVE EARLY!

Do not believe anything you have heard about the content of the cases from anyone!

Suggested Time Management

- Reading information on outside of door: *30 seconds*
- History: *8 minutes*
- Physical examination: *5 minutes*
- Closing and counseling: *2 minutes*
- Write-up: *10 minutes*

If you do not use the entire 15 minutes for the patient encounter and you leave early, the remaining time will be added to the time you have to write the Patient Note.

These are general guidelines *only*. If there is a lengthy description of the patient's reason for coming in, you may need more than 30 seconds to read it. Conversely, it may take you less time. Use common sense about how, when, and where to apply these guidelines or whether to deviate from them. Remember that these are just guidelines!

Types of Examination Cases

There are basically four types of examination cases. You will have 15 minutes to

- Perform a focused history and physical examination on the patient. When you enter the room, the patient will be undressed (underwear only) and in a hospital gown.
- Perform a focused history on the patient. This could also be the parent/guardian of a child who is not in the room. When you enter the room, the patient (or parent/guardian) will be dressed in street clothes. *Do not attempt to do a physical examination!*
- Counsel and/or educate the patient on a health-related issue (e.g., smoking cessation, safe sex, blood test results, weight reduction, biopsy results). The patient will be in street clothes.
- Do a telephone interview with a parent, guardian, care giver, or other individual such as an elderly individual. No one will be in the room when you enter.

The Patient Encounter

- Knock on the door before entering the room.
- Proper introduction sets the tone for the encounter.
- Identify yourself first. "*Hello, I am …*"
- Greet patient by his/her name. Always refer to the patient as "Mr.," "Mrs.," "Miss," "Dr.," or "Rev." If you are not told about the marital status of the woman, use the term "Ms." (pronounced "Miz") If you cannot pronounce the patient's name, ask him/her to pronounce it for you. This says more than how to call the patient; it tells the patient that you care for him/her as a person not a vehicle of disease! On the first visit, *never* call a patient by his/her first name even if they tell you it's okay. It changes the professional relationship to a more social one which is not good practice.
- Identify your role in the clinic.
- Inquire about comfort of the patient. Fix the patient's pillow or ask the patient if he/she is comfortable sitting or lying on the examination table.

- Use proper draping technique of the patient. Use the drape that is provided on the exam table or stool to cover the legs and knees of the patient to make the patient feel less exposed.
- Make comfortable eye contact.
- Keep your eye level generally at same level or below that of the patient (this depends on the position of the patient).
- Shake hands firmly (assuming that the patient does not have pain in the right hand/arm).
- Be pleasant and professional. A smile goes a long way in establishing rapport.

Treat *all* your encounters on this examination *exactly as you would treat any real patients* you may see with similar problems. Ask all the same questions and do whatever you feel necessary to do on the physical examination. The only exception is that you will *not* perform certain parts of the physical examination on any of the standardized patients, including the following:

Treat all your encounters on this examination exactly as you would treat any real patients you may see with similar problems.

- rectal
- internal pelvic
- genital or genitourinary
- female breast, or
- corneal reflex examinations

If you believe one or more of these examinations is/are indicated, you should include them in your proposed diagnostic workup in the Patient Note.

Ask any questions you wish and perform any part of the physical examination you consider pertinent. You will receive credit for anything that is on the patient checklist. There is *no* double jeopardy, that is, if you ask questions or perform physical examination techniques that are *not* on the checklist, you do *not* lose any credit—only time.

You should assume that you have consent to do a physical examination on all standardized patients unless you are explicitly told not to do so as part of the Examinee Instructions for that case. Although you want to be polite, you do not need to continually say, "Is that okay with you?"

Never undress your patient. Ask them to please untie or open their gown. If the patient is unable to do so because of weakness or arthritis, it is acceptable to say, "May I assist you in untying your gown?" In general, expose as little of the body as necessary and cover that part back up after examining it.

There is one blood pressure cuff which is the appropriate size for the patient in each room.

If the ophthalmoscope light is off, make sure that the on/off switch is illuminated. If not, switch it on by depressing the "I" button on the control. Also check that the dimmer switch is not set to low!

Never examine through a gown or article of clothing!

You must perform all physical examination maneuvers correctly. If an examination is not performed correctly, you will not receive credit for it! **Never examine through a gown or article of clothing!** There may or may not be positive physical findings present. Remember SPs are human beings and as such may really have diabetes with chronic stable diabetic retinopathy or heart murmurs. Some other findings may be simulated, but you should accept what you find as real and factor them into your evolving differential diagnoses. You must always attend to appropriate hygiene and to patient comfort and modesty, as you would in the care of real patients.

If there is a problem with equipment in the room, open the door and alert the proctor.

During the course of your physical examination, it is critical that you apply no more than the amount of pressure that is normally appropriate. This is especially important during maneuvers such as deep palpation of the abdomen; examination of the liver; carotid palpation; thyroid evaluation; eliciting costovertebral angle (CVA) tenderness; examination of the ears with the otoscope; reflex evaluation with the reflex hammer; and examination of the throat with the tongue depressor.

Remember to look at a patient's face for signs of possible pain when you perform the abdominal exam.

Synthetic models, mannequins, or simulators may be included to assess other examination skills such as those for the breast, pelvic, male genital, or rectal examinations.

Announcements During the Exam

There will be an announcement that will tell you when to begin the patient encounter. This is when you will slide the wooden panel to reveal the Examinee Instructions and begin to read them. *Never open the panel until instrusted to do so*. After you have read them, knock on the door and begin the encounter. When there are 5 minutes remaining, there will be an announcement, and another when the patient encounter is over. In some cases, you may complete the patient encounter in fewer than 15 minutes, although it is not advisable to do so. If so, you may leave the examination room early and begin the Patient Note, but you are not permitted to go back into the room. Because you cannot go back into the examination room, make sure that you have obtained all necessary information before leaving the room and don't forget to take your stethoscope. If you remember that you left your stethoscope in the room, tell the proctor who will get it for you.

The Patient Note

Immediately after each patient encounter, you will have 10 minutes to record a Patient Note. As noted above, if you leave the patient encounter early, you may use the additional time for the Patient Note. You will be asked to hand write or use a computer to write a Patient Note similar to a medical record you would write after seeing a patient. This normally includes the relevant pertinent positives and negatives of the medical history, the physical examination findings, your diagnostic impressions, and your plans for further evaluation.

The Step 2 CS Patient Note is a document of the patient's health history. The information that is recorded must be accurate and objective. On the basis of all the information gleaned from the patient's history and physical examination, the interviewer carefully summarizes all the data into a readable format. Only objective data should be included. Opinions or statements about previous care and therapy must be avoided.

By convention, all symptoms that the patient has experienced are indicated first. Symptoms never experienced are indicated afterward. The *pertinent positive symptoms/findings* are symptoms/findings that have possible relevance to the present illness and are presented first. *Pertinent negative symptoms/findings* are symptoms/findings that are not present but are often related to the present illness and are presented after the pertinent positive ones.

Pertinent positives always before pertinent negatives!

Always write *only* within the boxes provided. Any text handwritten outside the box will *not* be read. Because there is not much space, you may wish to use abbreviations. Use *only* those abbreviations that are listed in the USMLE Step 2 CS exam orientation materials, which are reprinted in Appendix A of this book. A copy of the abbreviations is also on the desk outside each room. It is always best to spell the word out if you are unsure whether the abbreviation is correct.

As long as the history and physical examination is comprehensible, you may use any style for writing it (e.g., prose, outline, bullets). Examples of different types of write-ups are included in the Patient Notes for the cases in Section IV of this book.

If you think a rectal, pelvic, genitourinary, female breast, or corneal reflex examination was indicated in the encounter, list it as part of your diagnostic workup. You will have five lines for the differential diagnosis and five lines for the diagnostic workup. Regarding blood tests, you must indicate the specific blood test needed (e.g., BUN [blood urea nitrogen], cholesterol, ALT [alanine aminotransferase], AST [aspartate aminotransferase], bilirubin, TSH [thyroid-stimulating hormone], T_3 [triiodothyronine], etc.) *and not*, for example, a comprehensive metabolic screen, liver function tests, or thyroid function tests. You are allowed to request a complete blood count (CBC) electrolytes, and urinalysis. All blood tests may be put on a single line.

If you think a rectal, pelvic, genitourinary, female breast, or corneal reflex examination was indicated in the encounter, list it as part of your diagnostic workup.

Hospitalization, treatment, consultations, or referrals cannot be included in your workup plan.

Hospitalization, treatment, consultations, or referrals cannot be included in your workup plan.

Figure 1 illustrates a blank patient note page similar to what you will be asked to complete if you write the note by hand. A program for practicing typing the patient note is available on the USMLE Orientation Materials CDROM and on the USMLE web site.

HISTORY

Include significant positives and negatives from history of present illness, past medical history, review of system(s), social history, and family history.

PHYSICAL EXAMINATION

Indicate only pertinent positive and negative findings related to the patient's chief complaint.

DIFFERENTIAL DIAGNOSES	DIAGNOSTIC WORKUP
In order of likelihood (with 1 being the most likely), list up to 5 potential or possible diagnoses for this patient's presentation (in many cases, fewer than 5 diagnoses are likely).	**List immediate plans (up to 5) for further diagnostic workup.**
1.	1.
2.	2.
3.	3.
4.	4.
5.	5.

Figure 1 Example of a Patient Note form should you elect to write it by hand. You are given an 8½ × 11-inch sheet of paper. The above example is reduced.

The Patient Note is another form of patient communication; it is communication sharing. Legibility counts! If your handwriting is difficult to read, you should probably print or use the computer to write your Patient Note.

It is important to know that if you choose to write your Patient Note by hand, do *not* touch any key on the keyboard because doing so will generate a blank patient note. If by accident you do touch the keyboard, notify a proctor immediately.

If you have a case for which you think no diagnostic workup is necessary, write "No studies indicated" rather than leaving that section blank. If you remember things that you should have asked or examination techniques that you forgot to do while in the patient room, *it is too late!* That's why it's important to stay in the room as long as possible.

Even if you plan to use the computer to write your Patient Note, make sure that your handwriting is legible. If the computer is not working for a specific station, you may be required to write that specific note by hand! Finally, practice writing a Patient Note in 10 minutes.

Although the physicians who read your notes have no knowledge of your particular SP encounters, they have extensive knowledge about each case they rate. However, you are cautioned to include only information obtained in your actual interview in the note; it is inappropriate to do otherwise.

When time is up, you will hear an announcement to stop writing. Put down your pen immediately or click "Submit" on the computer. Remain seated until the proctor has collected all the handwritten Patient Notes and the colored scrap paper that was used for that encounter.

There will be a Patient Note required after each encounter, including after the telephone interview. Because no physical examination is possible, it is acceptable to leave that section of the Patient Note blank or indicate what you would do when you would see the patient.

Include only information in your Patient Note that you obtained in your actual interview or physical exam!

When time is up for writing the Patient Note, put down your pen immediately *or click "Submit" on the computer.*

Important Web Sites

AAMC	Association of American Medical Colleges http://www.aamc.org
AMA	American Medical Association http://www.ama-assn.org
ACGME	Accreditation Council for Graduate Medical Education http://www.acgme.org
ERAS	The Electronic Residency Application Service http://www.aamc.org/audienceeras.htm
FSMB	Federation of State Medical Boards http://www.fsmb.org

NRMP National Resident Matching Program
http://www.nrmp.org

OASIS On-Line Applicant Status and Information System
https://oasis2.ecfmg.org

USMLE United States Medical Licensing Examination
http://www.usmle.org

Always check the USMLE (www.usmle.org) and ECFMG (www.ecfmg.org) web sites frequently for the latest information about the exam.

Finally, always check the USMLE (www.usmle.org) and ECFMG (www.ecfmg.org) web sites frequently for the latest information about the exam.

Section 2

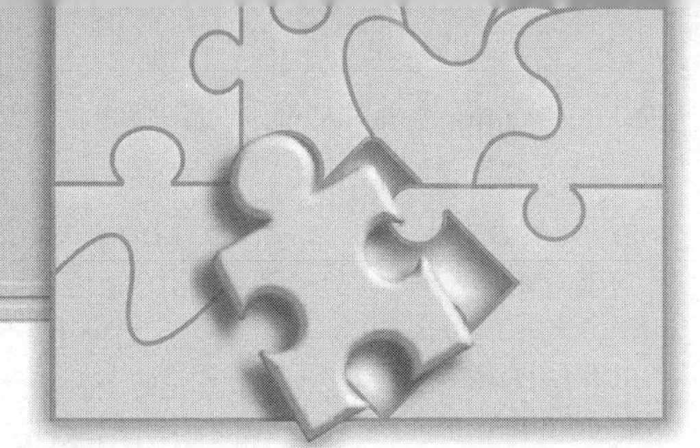

Communication Skills

General Principles

Interviewing, by its very nature, is dynamic and everchanging. Because it cannot be reduced to a preconceived set of guidelines or algorithms, all the following suggestions are just that—suggestions. The conversation that occurs between a patient and physician is a unique and private one that cannot be predicted. The facilitating tools outlined here, however, can be applied in most situations.

The conversation that occurs between a patient and physician is a unique and private one that cannot be predicted.

Good communication skills are the foundation of excellent medical care. Even with the exciting new technology that has appeared in the last decade, excellent communicative behavior is still paramount in the care of patients. Studies show that good communication improves patient outcomes by resolving symptoms and reducing patients' psychological distress and anxiety.

The main purpose of an interview is to gather all basic information pertinent to the patient's illness and the patient's adaptation to illness. An assessment of the patient's condition can then be made. An experienced interviewer considers all the aspects of the patient's presentation and follows the leads that appear to deserve the most attention.

Any patient who seeks consultation from a clinician needs to be evaluated in the broadest sense. The clinician must be keenly aware of all clues, obvious or subtle. Although body language is important, the spoken word remains the central diagnostic tool in medicine. For this reason, the art of speaking and listening continues to be the central part of the doctor–patient interaction. Once all the clues from the history have been gathered, the assimilation of those clues into an ultimate diagnosis is relatively easy.

Communication is the key to a successful interview. The interviewer must be able to ask questions of the patient freely. These questions must always be easily understood and adjusted to the medical sophistication of the patient. If necessary, slang words describing certain conditions may be used to facilitate communication and avoid misunderstanding.

The best interview is conducted by an interviewer who is cheerful, friendly, and genuinely concerned about the patient.

The best interview is conducted by an interviewer who is cheerful, friendly, and genuinely concerned about the patient.

In the beginning, the patient will most likely bring up the subjects that are easiest to discuss. More painful experiences can be elicited by tactful questioning. The novice interviewer needs to gain experience to feel comfortable asking questions about subjects that are more painful, delicate, or unpleasant. Timing of such questions is critical.

A cardinal principle of interviewing is to permit patients to express their stories in their own words. The manner in which patients tell their stories reveals much about the nature of their illnesses. Careful observation of a patient's facial expressions and body movements may provide valuable nonverbal clues. The interviewer may also use body language such as a smile, nod, silence, hand gesture, or a questioning look to encourage the patient to continue the story.

Listening without interruption is important and requires skill.

Listening without interruption is important and requires skill. If given the chance, patients often disclose their problems spontaneously. Interviewers need to *hear* what is being said. Allow the patient to finish his/her answer, even if there are pauses while the patient processes his or her feelings. All too often, an interview may fail to reveal all the clues because the interviewer did not take the time to allow the patient to speak and did not listen to the patient.

Listen more, talk less, and interrupt infrequently.

The best clinical interview focuses on the patient, not on the clinician's agenda. An important rule for improved interviewing is *to listen more, talk less, and interrupt infrequently*. Interrupting disrupts the patient's train of thought. Allow the patient, at least in part, to control the interview.

Interviewers should be attentive to how patients use their words to conceal or reveal their thoughts and history. Interviewers should be wary of quick, very positive statements such as, "Everything's fine," "I'm very happy," or "No problems." If interviewers have reason to doubt these statements, they may respond by saying, "Is everything really as fine as it could be?"

If the history given is vague, the interviewer may use direct questioning. Asking "how," "where," or "when" is generally more effective than asking "why," which tends to put patients on the defensive. Try asking "What is the reason ..." instead of "Why ..."

Always treat the patient with respect. Do not contradict or impose your moral standards on the patient.

The interviewer must be able to question patients about subjects that may be distressing or embarrassing to the interviewer, the patient, or both. Because answers to many routine questions may cause embarrassment to interviewers and leave them speechless, interviewers tend to avoid such questions. The interviewer's ability to be open and frank about such topics promotes the likelihood of discussion in those areas.

Very often, patients feel comfortable discussing what an interviewer would consider antisocial behavior, such as drug addiction, or "aberrations" of sexual behavior. Interviewers must be careful not to pass judgment on this "unusual" behavior.

A broad interest in body language has evolved. This type of nonverbal communication, in association with spoken language, can provide a more total picture of the patient's behavior. Biting of ones nails, shaking the hand or foot, articles of clothing, or playing with or removing a wedding band[1] can provide additional information about the patient. Use your eyes to see!

Touching the patient can also be very useful. Touch can communicate warmth, affection, caring, and understanding. Many factors, including gender and cultural background, as well as the location of the touch, influence the response to the touch. Touching on a shoulder for about 2 seconds is generally the best way of demonstrating this caring.

Touch can communicate warmth, affection, caring, and understanding.

A good interviewing session determines what the patient understands about their own health problems. What does the *patient* think is wrong with them? This is always an important question to ask a patient. It can lead nowhere or can provide valuable information about the patient's anxiety about their illness and their level of medical knowledge.

What does the patient think is wrong with them?

If during the interview you cannot answer a question, do not. You can always act as the patient's advocate; listen to the question and then find someone who can provide an appropriate answer. Although you may not be able to answer the question, assure the patient that you will research it and get back to them with the proper resource or answer.

A very important task of communication is to engage the patient. A helpful way of building rapport with your patient who is not acutely ill is to be curious about the person as a whole. Ask, "Before we begin, tell me something about yourself."

Federal Health Information Privacy Law

Before your examination, it is important to review the **HIPAA regulations** (Health Insurance Portability and Accountability Act (HIPAA) of 1996): www.hhs.gov/ocr/hipaa. This is a federal law that protects the privacy of a patient's health information. This law sets the rules and limits on who can look at and receive patient information. A patient's health information cannot be used or shared without the written permission of the patient. Without this permission, the health care provider cannot

- give health information to an employer;
- use or share information for marketing of advertising purposes;
- share private notes about a patient's mental health counseling sessions.

[1]A patient who is removing a wedding band may be telling you by body language that they are unhappy with their marriage. Be curious and inquire about their relationship.

Physicians, nurses, pharmacies, clinics, nursing homes, and other health care providers must follow this law in addition to health insurance companies and health maintenance organizations (HMOs).

Conducting the Interview

You should make the patient as comfortable as possible. If the patient's eyeglasses, hearing aids, or dentures were removed, ask whether he or she would like to use them.

The interviewer should introduce him/herself, greet the patient by their last name, make eye contact, shake hands firmly, and smile. The interviewer may wish to say,

> "Good morning, I'm Mary Jones, a medical student at the … School of Medicine. I've been asked to interview and examine you in the next 15 minutes. Are you Mr. Smith? Did I pronounce your name correctly"

Or if appropriate,

> "Good morning, I'm Dr. Jones, a staff doctor here at the medical center (clinic). I've been asked to interview and examine you in the next 15 minutes. Are you Mr. Smith? Did I pronounce your name correctly"

The information on the Examinee Instructions will let you know who you are in relationship to the patient. Read it carefully!

Always introduce yourself first before pronouncing the patient's name. It is also correct to ask the patient how to pronounce their name.

Do not address the patient by his/her first name, even if they say it is okay.

When introducing yourself to a patient, always say your name slowly. You know your name, but the patient doesn't. It is not important to use your first name. But it is important to pause between the word "Dr." and your last name. *"Hi, I am Dr. . . . Jones."* The pause is important because the "r" of doctor often runs into the last name, rendering it difficult to understand.

It is appropriate to address patients by their correct titles—Mr., Mrs., Dr., Rev., Ms.—unless they are adolescents or younger. *Do not address the patient by his/her first name, even if they say it is okay.* Once on a first name basis, you have changed the doctor–patient relationship to a more informal setting!

Normally, the interviewer and patient should be seated comfortably at the same level. Sometimes it is useful to have the patient sitting even higher than the interviewer to give the patient the visual advantage.

Regardless of whether the patient is sitting in a chair or lying in bed, make sure that the patient is appropriately draped with a sheet or robe if they are undressed.

Once the introduction has been made, you may begin the interview by asking a general, open-ended question, such as *"What medical problem has brought you to the hospital?"*

Novice interviewers are often worried about remembering the patient's history. It is poor form to write extensive notes during the interview. Attention should be focused more on what the person is saying and less on the written word.

After the introductory question, the interviewer should proceed to questions related to the chief complaint. These should naturally evolve into questions related to the other formal parts of the medical history, such as the present illness, past illnesses, social and family history, and review of body systems.

Small talk (i.e., talking about the weather or if the patient had any problem coming to see you) is a useful method of enhancing the narrative.

When patients use vague terms such as "often," "somewhat," "a little," "fair," "reasonably well," "sometimes," "rarely," or "average," the interviewer must always ask for clarification.

You should be alert for subtle clues from the patient that will guide your interview further. For example, hesitation in answering a question, or looking away from you, staring at you, or fidgeting are indications that there is something else going on that bears further inquiry.

You should be alert for subtle clues from the patient that will guide your interview further.

The interviewer may wish to summarize for the patient the most important parts of the history to help illuminate the significant points made.

At the conclusion, it is polite to encourage the patient to discuss any additional problems or to ask any questions. *"Is there anything else you would like to tell me that I have not already asked?" "Are there any questions you might like to ask?"*

Remember that when interviewing real patients by using direct questions, most of the answers will be "No." Do not become upset on this exam when the same is true. If these questions are important to ask, they are pertinent negatives and will be on the checklists!

Basic Interviewing Techniques

Questioning

Open-Ended Questions

Open-ended questions are used to ask the patient for general information. This type of question is most useful in opening up the interview or for changing the topic to be discussed. An open-ended question allows the patient to tell his or her story spontaneously and does not presuppose a specific answer. An open-ended question cannot be answered by a one-word answer. It can be useful to allow the patient to "ramble on." Allow patients at least 15 to 20 seconds to answer before you cut them off and refocus the dialogue. If the patient is telling you pertinent information, it may not be necessary to cut them off at all! Examples of open-ended questions are the following:

"What kind of medical problem are you having?"
"How has your health been?"
"Are you having stomach pain? Tell me about it."

Direct Questions

After a period of open-ended questioning, the interviewer needs to direct the questioning to specific facts learned during the open-ended questioning period. These direct questions serve to clarify and add detail to the story. This type of question gives the patient little room for explanation or qualification. A direct question can usually be answered in one word or a brief sentence. For example,

"Where does it hurt?"
"When do you get the burning?"

BODILY LOCATION

"Where in your back?"
"Can you tell me where you feel the pain?"

ONSET (CHRONOLOGY)

"When did you first notice it?"
"How long did it last?"

PRECIPITATING FACTORS

"What makes it worse?"
"What seems to bring on the pain?"

PALLIATING FACTORS

"What do you do to get more comfortable?"
"Does lying quietly in bed help you?"

QUALITY

"What does it feel like?"
"Can you describe the pain?""

RADIATION

"When you get the pain in your chest, do you feel it in any other part of your body?"

SEVERITY

"On a scale from 1 to 10, with 10 the worst pain you can imagine, how would you rate this pain?"
"How has the pain affected your lifestyle?"

TEMPORAL

"Does it ever occur at rest?"
"Does the pain occur when you are hungry?"
"Does the pain occur with your menstrual cycle?"

ASSOCIATED MANIFESTATIONS

"Do you ever have nausea with the pain?"
"Have you noticed other changes that happen when you start to sweat?"

The mnemonic **O-P-Q-R-S-T**, which stands for *o*nset (chronology), *p*recipitating (and *p*alliative), *q*uality, *r*adiation, *s*everity, and *t*emporal, is useful to help you remember these important dimensions of a symptom.

The mnemonic **O-P-Q-R-S-T**, which stands for *o*nset (chronology), *p*recipitating (and *p*alliative), *q*uality, *r*adiation, *s*everity, and *t*emporal, is useful to help you remember these important dimensions of a symptom.

Question Types to Avoid

There are several types of questions that should be avoided. One is the **suggestive question**, which provides the answer to the question. For example,

"Do you feel the pain in your left arm when you get it in your chest?"

A better way to ask the same question would be,

"When you get the pain in your chest, do you notice it anywhere else?"

The ***"Why"* question** carries tones of accusation. This type of question almost always asks a patient to account for his or her behavior and tends to put the person on the defensive. For example,

"Why did you stop taking the medication?"

The answers, however, to the "Why" question are important. Try rephrasing the "why" question to "What is the reason…?"

"What is the reason you haven't seen a doctor for three years?"

The **multiple or rapid-fire question** should also be avoided. In this type of question, there is more than one point of inquiry. Don't barrage the patient with a list of questions. The patient can easily get confused and respond incorrectly, answering no part of the question adequately. The patient may answer only the last inquiry heard. More importantly, you may feel like you have asked the question and received an answer when really you have not! For example,

"Have you had night sweats, fever, or chills?"

The patient may answer, *"No"* but was answering only about the chills. It is preferable to ask, *"Do you have night sweats?" "Do you have a fever?" "Have you had chills?"*

Questions should be concise and easily understood. The context should be **free of medical jargon**. For example,

"You seem to have a homonymous hemianopsia."
"Have you ever had a myocardial infarction?"

are examples of bad questions to ask.

Ask patients to describe what they mean when they use medical jargon. For example, some patients may use "heart attack" to describe angina, "stroke" to describe a transient ischemic attack, "spells" to describe dizziness, or "water pills" or "heart pills" when referring to their medication.

A **leading or biased question** carries a suggestion of the kind of response for which the interviewer is looking. As an example,

"You haven't used any recreational drugs, have you?"
"You don't have asthma, do you?"

It is better to ask,

> "Do you use recreational drugs?"
> "Do you have asthma?"

Be careful not to phrase your questions negatively!

Therefore, be careful not to phrase your questions negatively!

Always avoid **false assurances**. *"We'll definitely make you feel better"* is a false assurance. It is better to say, *"We will do everything possible to make you feel better."* False assurances restore a patient's confidence but ignore the reality of the situation.

Table 1 reviews examples of questions to avoid.

Never assume anything about a patient's knowledge of their disease, their sexual orientation or experiences, their education, their family, or their knowledge of illness in general. Your patient will always surprise you by knowing more or less about a particular topic. This is particularly true in counseling cases.

Silence

This technique is most useful with silent patients. Silence should never be used with overtalkative patients, because letting them "have the floor" does not allow the interviewer to control the interview.

Facilitation

Facilitation is a technique of verbal or nonverbal communication that encourages a patient to continue speaking but does not direct the patient to a topic. A common verbal facilitation is *"Uh huh."* Other examples of verbal facilitations include *"Go on," "Tell me more about that," "And then?,"* and *"Hmm."*

TABLE 1. **Examples of Question Types to Avoid**

	Incorrect Question	Preferred Question
Suggestive Question	"Do you have pain in your shoulder when you get it in your abdomen?"	"When you get the pain in your abdomen, do you notice it anywhere else?"
"Why" Question	"Why did you come in to see me today when you've had the pain for 3 weeks?"	"What is the reason you came in today after having the pain for 3 weeks?"
Multiple Question	"Have you had nausea, vomiting, or diarrhea?"	"Did you have nausea? "Have you been throwing up?" "Have you had diarrhea?"
Technical Jargon	"Have you ever had a CVA?"	"Have you ever had a stroke?"
Leading Question	"You're not gay, are you?" "You don't have shortness of breath, do you?" "You don't have heart disease, do you?"	"Are you gay?" "Do you have a history of shortness of breath?" "Do you have heart disease?"
False Assurance	"I'll give you some pain medications so you will definitely not have any pain."	"I'll do everything possible to help you."

An important nonverbal facilitation is nodding the head or making a hand gesture to continue. Moving toward the patient connotes interest. Be careful not to nod too much, as this may convey approval in situations in which approval might not be intended.

Another technique is to simply repeat back to the patient what they have just said. This indicates to the patient that you have really been listening to them and heard what they have said.

Confrontation

Confrontation is a response based on an observation by the interviewer that points out something striking about the patient's behavior or previous statement. This interviewing technique directs the patient's attention to something of which the patient may or may not be aware. The confrontation may be either a statement or a question. For example,

"You look upset."
"What is the reason you are not answering my questions?"

Confrontation is particularly useful in encouraging the patient to continue the narrative when there are subtle clues given. Confrontation must be used with care; excessive use is considered impolite and overbearing. If correctly used, however, confrontation can be a powerful technique.

Interpretation

Interpretation is a type of confrontation that is based on inference rather than on observation. The interviewer must fully understand the clues the patient has given before the interviewer can offer an interpretation. Examples are the following:

"You seem to be quite happy about that."
"Sounds like you're scared."

Support

Support is a response that indicates an interest in or an understanding of the patient. Supportive remarks promote a feeling of security in the doctor–patient relationship. *Support or empathy is vital to be shown with all patients, especially on the Step 2 CS exam!* A supportive response might be, *"Tell me how I can help"* or *"This must be very difficult for you."* Be careful, however, about saying *"I understand."* Especially with hostile patients, this can backfire with the patient confronting you.

Support or empathy is vital to be shown with all patients, especially on the Step 2 CS exam!

You should also be careful about saying, *"Relax," "Don't worry,"* or *"Don't cry."* Allow the patient to respond in whatever way the patient needs. If your patient begins to cry, it is acceptable to offer a box of tissues.

Two important subgroups of support are *assurance* and *empathy*. An example of assurance is the following:

"That's wonderful! I'm delighted that you started in the rehabilitation program at the hospital."
"Congratulations on stopping smoking! That's a big achievement."

Examples of empathy are the following:

"I'm sure your daughter's problem has given you much anxiety."
"You must have been very sad."

Transitions

Transitional statements are used as guides to allow the patient to understand better the logic of your questioning and for the interview to flow more smoothly from one topic to another. An example of a transitional statement might be, after learning about the current medical problem, your stating,

"Now I am going to ask you some questions about your past medical history."

Other examples are:

"Okay, now let's talk about your lifestyle and your activities in a typical day."
"I am now going to ask you some routine questions about your sexual history."

Avoid phrases such as "personal habits" or "personal history" because these expressions send the message of what the interviewer considers these habits to be.

Avoid words such as "like," "have to," or "want to."

Also avoid words such as "like," "have to," or "want to." It is preferable to say, "I am going to." For example, *"I am going to do a chest exam"* instead of *"I would like to do a chest exam."*

Format of the History

Just listen to your patient and follow their leads.

The information obtained by the interviewer is organized traditionally into a comprehensive statement about the patient's health. **On Step 2 CS, it is very likely that you will not be able to ask all these questions because of the 15-minute time limit. Just listen to your patient and follow their leads. Go with their directions—not yours! Do not feel compelled to ask all the questions in these divisions of the history. The patient's initial responses to your open-ended questions will steer you toward those questions you need to ask.**

A word about mnemonics—use them sparingly! If you have no problem remembering what the letters mean, you can use them, but all too often you will remember the letters of the mnemonic but forget what they stand for. During a written or computer test, no one is looking at your face while you are trying to remember what the letters indicate; this exam is quite different. You might want to jot down a mnemonic you find useful on the scrap paper before you enter the room; if you run out of things to ask, look at the mnemonic for help.

The major traditional sections of the history are as follows:

- Source and reliability
- Chief complaint
- History of the present illness and debilitating symptoms
- Past medical history
- Health maintenance
- Occupational and environmental history
- Biographic information
- Family history
- Psychosocial and spiritual history
- Sexual, reproductive, and gynecologic history
- Review of systems

Source and Reliability

The source is usually the patient, although in the case of a telephone encounter or a pediatric encounter, it is sometimes a care giver. The reliability of the interview should be assessed early in the interview, especially in patients older than 65 years of age, by checking orientation to person, time, and place.

Chief Complaint

The chief complaint (CC) is the patient's brief statement explaining why he or she sought medical attention. In the written history, it is frequently a quoted statement of the patient, such as

"Chest pain for the past 5 hours."
"Terrible nausea and vomiting for 2 days."

History of Present Illness and Debilitating Symptoms

The history of the present illness (HPI) refers to the recent changes in health that led the patient to seek medical attention at this time. It describes the information relevant to the chief complaint. It should answer the questions what, when, how, where, which, who, and what is the reason.

Past Medical History

The past medical history (PMH) consists of the overall assessment of the patient's health before the present illness. **You will probably not have the time to ask all the questions in these areas for any one patient on the Step 2 CS exam**. The PMH includes all of the following:

- General state of health
- Past illnesses
- Injuries
- Hospitalizations
- Surgery
- Allergies
- Immunizations
- Substance abuse (caffeine, nicotine, alcohol, recreational drugs, other agents)
- Diet, appetite, weight gain/loss
- Sleep patterns
- Current medications
- Complementary and alternative therapies

As an **introduction** to the past medical history, the interviewer may ask,

"How has your health been in the past?"

When asking about **hospitalizations**, you can ask,

"Have you ever been hospitalized?

Patients will generally indicate hospitalizations for medical or surgical illnesses. However, patients may not tell you about hospitalizations for psychiatric illnesses. If you suspect psychiatric hospitalizations, follow the first question with,

"Have you ever been hospitalized for non-medical or non-surgical reasons?"

Always ask about allergies.

Always ask about **allergies**. If a patient has an allergy, find out how they know they have an allergy and what happens to them (e.g., rash, anaphylaxis).

Don't forget about the **CAGE questionnaire** for any person with possible alcohol or recreational drug use.

C – cut down

A – annoyed

G – guilty

E – "eye opener"

Related to **medications**, ask the following four questions:

- "Do you use prescription medications?"
- "Do you use over-the-counter medications?"
- "Do you use herbal medications?"
- "Do you use recreational drugs?"

Health Maintenance

Physicians can play a key role in the identification and management of medical, social, and psychiatric problems. Counseling skills include building a supportive therapeutic relationship with the patient and family. A patient's family can often be helpful in confirming the diagnosis and developing the treatment plan. Health maintenance consists of three main areas: disease detection, disease prevention, and health promotion. *This is very important on Step 2 CS; don't forget to ask about it!*

Ask patients whether they have regular doctors and routine medical checkups. When was their last dental examination? Do they get their eyes checked periodically? Are they aware of their cholesterol levels? Do they do anything for exercise?

If the patient is a woman, does she see a gynecologist regularly? Does she do breast self-examination? When was her last mammogram and her last Papanicolaou (Pap) smear? If the patient is a man, does he do routine testicular self-examination?

Occupational and Environmental History

The occupational and environmental history concerns exposure to potential disease-producing substances or environments. The following are some of the questions regarding occupational and environmental exposure that could be asked:

"What type of work do you do?"
"How long have you been doing this work?"
"Describe your work."
"Are you exposed to any hazardous materials? Do you ever use protective equipment?"
"What kind of work did you do before you had your present job?"
"Have you ever lived near any factories, shipyards, or other potentially hazardous facilities?"
"Has anyone in your household ever worked with hazardous materials that could have been brought home?"
"What types of hobbies do you have? What types of exposures are involved?"
"Do you now or have you previously had environmental or occupational exposure to asbestos, lead, fumes, chemicals, dusts, loud noise, radiation, or other toxic factors?"

Biographic Information

Biographic information includes the date and place of birth, sex, race, and ethnic background.

Family History

The family history provides information about the health of the entire family—living and dead. Pay particular attention to possible genetic and environmental aspects of disease that might have implications for the patient. You can start this section by asking,

"Tell me a little about your family."
"Are your parents alive?"
"How is their health?"

Psychosocial and Spiritual History

The psychosocial history includes information on the education, life experiences, and personal relationships of the patient. This section should include the patient's lifestyle, other people living with the patient, schooling, military service, religious beliefs (in relation to the perceptions of health and treatment), and marital or significant-other relationships. You can start by asking:

"Tell me a little about yourself—your background, education, work, and family."
"Who lives at home with you?"
"Who are the important people in your life?"
"How do you feel about the way your life is going?"

These are important questions but may not need to be asked of all your patients.

Sexual, Reproductive, and Gynecologic History

Anxiety, depression, and anger may relate to sexual dysfunction.

There are several reasons for taking a sexual history. Sexual drive is a sensitive indicator of general well-being. Anxiety, depression, and anger may relate to sexual dysfunction; however, many physical symptoms can lead to sexual problems. In addition, it is critical to identify risk behaviors. A well-taken sexual history enables the examiner to establish norms of sexuality for the patient. Opening up the interview to issues of sexuality allows the interviewer to educate the patient about human immunodeficiency virus (HIV)-related illnesses, sexually transmitted diseases, and pregnancy prevention. It is an excellent opportunity to provide useful information to the patient. ***It is a very important part of your communication skills that are assessed on Step 2 CS!***

There are several general questions that can help broach the topic of sexual activity. Start by asking, *"Are you sexually active?"* If the answer is *"No,"* ask, *"Have you ever been sexually active?"* If the answer is *"Yes,"* ask, *"Are your partners male, female, or both?"* Some of the following questions might also be helpful.

> "Are you having any sexual problems?"
> "Are you satisfied with your sexual performance?" "Do you think your partner is?" If not, "What is unsatisfactory to you (or your partner)?"
> "Have you had any difficulty achieving orgasm?"
> "Are there any questions pertaining to your sexual performance that you would like to discuss?"
> "Do you have protected sex?"
> "Have you ever had a sexually transmitted disease?"
> "Have you been tested for HIV?" If yes, "What was the result?"

Do not cast judgment on a patient's answers to their sexual habits.

Review of Systems

The review of systems summarizes in terms of body systems all the symptoms that may have been overlooked in the history of the present illness or in the medical history. By reviewing in an orderly manner the list of possible symptoms, the interviewer can specifically check each system and uncover additional symptoms of "unrelated" illnesses not yet discussed. The review of systems is best organized from the head down to the extremities, and the questions can be asked while the physical examination of that body area is being examined.

After the History—Before the Physical Examination

Do not give false assurances.

- Summarize the patient's condition. This tells the patient that you were listening to the story and allows the patient to correct it!
- Do not give false assurances.
- End with a statement such as, *"Is there anything else that you would like to tell me that I have not already asked?"* or *"Do you have any questions for me?"*
- Thank the patient and tell the patient that you are going to wash your hands before you begin the physical examination.

Specific Patient Challenges

"I'm in pain."

Show *empathy* by stating that you see that the person is very uncomfortable and you will give the patient pain medications as soon as possible.

Tell the patient you still need to do an examination, which you will do as quickly as possible and as gently as possible. Once you know what is wrong, you will then provide the patient with something to make him/her more comfortable.

The Noncooperative Patient

Most of these patients are afraid. Try to assure them that they are in "good hands" and try to allay their fears about their illness if possible.

"Will the Test Hurt?"

As above, most of these patients are more fearful about the possibility of disease and the outcome of the test than about the test itself. Educate the patient about the importance of the test. If you know that a certain test will hurt, educate the patient about its importance. *Remember, Step 2 CS is an assessment of your communication skills!*

"Am I Going to Die?"

Patients asking this question are really asking "*How* will they die?" Will they die with pain? Will they die alone? Assure the patient that you will do everything possible to provide them with relief from pain, and that you will be with them to support them in any way you can.

"Do I Have Cancer?"

In most cases, you can always answer that it is too premature to answer that question without the benefit of blood studies and other tests. Once you get the results, you will be in a better position to answer that question. In some cases, when pushed by the patient, you may have to state, *"Yes, you may have cancer, but there are many other things it could be. Let's get the test results first and then we can discuss it."*

The Geriatric Patient

The geriatric patient presents a special problem because in this patient, the emphasis is more on *function* and less on diagnosis. In any patient age 65 years or older, always test for orientation to person, time, and place, and ask about the activities of daily living (ADL)

Dressing
Eating
Ambulating
Toileting
Hygiene

as well as the instrumental activities of daily living (IADL)

Shopping
Housekeeping

Accounting
Food preparation
Transportation/telephone

Closure

After completing the physical examination, it is **vital** to provide some closure to the encounter. You are expected to summarize the findings and provide some general statement of the patient's condition. In most cases, you will not be able to provide a diagnosis as the complaint is often so broad (e.g., headache, back pain, fatigue). In addition, without test results, it is often nearly impossible to provide a single diagnosis. *Remember, this exam is not assessing your ability to make a diagnosis; it is an assessment of your ability to communicate!*

Remember, this exam is not assessing your ability to make a diagnosis; it is an assessment of your ability to communicate!

You may be able to suggest a diagnostic workup and discuss that with the patient. You should try to answer any questions the patient might have. If you don't know an answer to a question, be honest and say, "I don't know." It's okay to comment that you will find out the answer and get back to them.

It is also appropriate to say, "Have you understood everything we discussed today?" Then ask, "Do you have any anything else that you would like to discuss today?" Reassure the patient that they will be well taken care of. And, finally, say, "Thank you very much. Please do not hesitate to call me again if you have any questions."

If time is up, at the very least *always* spend 5 seconds more just to say that you have been called away for an emergency but you will return as soon as possible to answer any questions. Then quickly leave the room.

Common Exam Mistakes

Some of the more common examination mistakes are as follows:

- Not fully understanding the objectives of the examination.
- Not reading the Examinee Instructions carefully. Everything that is described is pertinent!
- Thinking that you have to pass every case in order to pass the exam. In fact, it is possible to pass the exam if you have done poorly on a few cases but very well on others.
- Poor time management.
- Not listening to the patient and following the patient's leads.
- Using your "list" or your agenda.
- Interrupting the patient and not listening to the patient's answer to your question.

Just move on to the next room and do not let your feelings about a previous encounter jeopardize your next encounter(s)!

- Becoming flustered by the patient's attitude, challenges, or questions.
- Leaving the room too early, or wasting time before entering the room.
- Giving the patient a premature diagnosis.
- Trying to reconstruct what just happened in the room after the encounter; you should just move on to the next room and do not let your feelings about a previous encounter jeopardize your next encounter(s)!
- Forgetting that the USMLE is looking to see how you would act in a real clinic environment.
- Not taking the encounter seriously

Listen to everything that is said and observe all body language!

Believe it or not, the standardized patients are rooting for you to pass the exam!

Be aware of everything that happens during a specific scenario; nothing is extraneous. Listen to everything that is said and observe all body language! It is true that the standardized patients (SPs) are there to give you a hard time and provide many communication challenges, but they are *not* there to fail you! Believe it or not, they are rooting for you to pass the exam! The SPs are constantly providing clues, which if you hear and see them, will help you to ask the appropriate questions and gather all the data necessary.

If you think that you did not do well on an encounter, take a deep breath, stretch, shake off the "bad" encounter, take another deep breath, and start your next one with a smile.

Spoken English Proficiency (for the International Medical Graduate)

Speak Slowly and Enunciate Clearly

It is most important to speak more slowly than you would during casual conversation; make sure that your patient comprehends what you are saying. Certain cultures have a tendency to speak fast and, thus, their English also tends to be fast. It is critically important, especially if you are not a native English speaker and you have a thick accent, to speak slowly and enunciate clearly. Choose simple words and keep your sentences short! Use few adjectives and adverbs! Practice listening to radio and television. Practice speaking with a native English speaker.

Volume

The volume of your spoken voice is also important. *Be strong,* but not overpowering in your volume. Patients like a strong voice that conveys confidence.

Acknowledge Your Accent

If you do have a thick accent, acknowledge it! It is fine to say that English is not your first language and you are speaking slowly so that the patient will comprehend what you are saying. If you have difficulty thinking about what to say or ask and there is a pause, merely say, "*Please give me a moment to think.*"

Introduce Your Own Name First

It is best that you begin the entire scenario by introducing *yourself* first, and then ask the patient how to pronounce their name. It is not necessary to use your first, or given, name. This introduction occurs within the critical first 5 seconds of the interview, and you do not want to start off on the wrong foot by pronouncing the patient's name incorrectly!

Choose Your Words Carefully

There are several words that non-native English speakers frequently have trouble pronouncing. It is often difficult to pronounce words beginning with a "*v*" such as "*vomit;*" use the synonym "*throw up*" instead. Instead of asking a patient to spell the word "*world,*" ask them to spell the word "*earth.*" It's easier to say.

Problematic Words and Expressions

One problematic word is "*abortion.*" Abortion in many parts of the world is used synonymously to mean an ending of a pregnancy or a miscarriage. In the United States, abortion is a very emotionally charged word. The word "*miscarriage*" is better than "*abortion*" and does not carry the same emotional weight as "*abortion.*" When taking an obstetrical history from a woman, it is preferable to ask, "*What was the outcome of the pregnancy (or pregnancies)?*"

In United Kingdom-trained physicians, the word "motions" is commonly used to ask about defecation. In the United States, the correct expression is "bowel movements." Also the terms "front passage" and "back passage" are not used in the United States.

Unless you are speaking to a child, the word "tummy" is better replaced with either the word "abdomen" or "stomach."

Words to Practice Pronunciation

The following words may present difficulties to non-native English speakers. It would be useful, therefore, to find a source (e.g., radio, television, English language courses, or native English speakers) for the proper pronunciation of the following words and then practice saying them:

urgent, voice, neighbor, lifelong, anymore, apparently, practically, complicated, worse, seem, progress, missed, anything, loose, approximately, Alzheimer's, ask, barbiturate, breathe, breath, breast, clothes, other, nuclear, often, prescription, prostate, diphtheria, height

There are also some English words that have silent letters and are commonly mispronounced. These include

calm, climb, could, doubt, half, herb, herbal, honest, hour, knowledge, muscle, psychology, should, subtle, talk, walk

TOEFL (Test of English as a Foreign Language)

If you would like to ascertain whether your spoken English is acceptable for the exam, take the TOEFL (Test of English as a Foreign Language) examination. A score of 35 or higher is probably acceptable for taking Step 2 CS. The TOEFL is no longer a requirement for taking Step 2 CS, but it may provide some guidance as to whether your English might be a problem for the exam. For more information, you might want to contact:

TOEFL
P.O. Box 6151
Princeton, NJ 08541-6151
(609) 771-7100
www.toefl.org

In Summary

Always remember:

- Listen more
- Talk less
- Interrupt infrequently

A medical history must be dynamic. Every history is different. All patients may be asked the standard questions, but each patient should be evaluated individually. There is no limit to the questions to be asked.

If you find yourself lost, tell the patient that you would like to summarize or review what they have told you. This will allow you to take a deep breath, look over any notes, and get back on track.

In Closing

I hope the information in this section will prove useful for you on the exam, as well as enhance the quality of your patient encounters for the duration of your medical career. Good luck on the exam!

Section 3

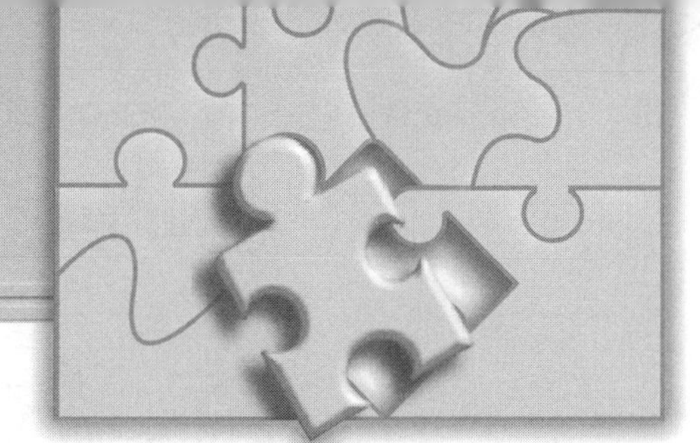

As "American" As Apple Pie—A Brief Cultural Guide

AMERICAN CULTURE

The United States developed from colonies owned primarily by the British, French, Dutch, and, later, Spanish Empires. It was formed following the Declaration of Independence from England in 1776. Today, the American culture continues to be a melting pot with great diversity and strong influences from Europeans, Native Americans, African-Americans, Asians, and other immigrants. The government is a federal republic system with free elections. The President of the United States is both Chief of State and Head of the Government; the term is for four years.

Because of the great diversity of the United States, there isn't a single "American style." The Northeast is different from the South which is different from the Midwest, which is different from the cultural attitude of the West. Lifestyles, food, and culture tend to differ within different areas. In general, however, Americans enjoy individualism, altruism, equality, democracy, Judeo-Christian morals, and patriotism, to name a few ideals.

In the United States, there are federal, state, and local laws. Federal laws apply to the entire country. State laws include driving speeds, sales tax, etc., and are passed by the state legislature and signed into law by the state governor. These state laws exist under or parallel to federal laws. State laws can be stronger than federal laws (e.g., a state minimum wage can be higher than the federal minimum wage), but they cannot weaken or be less stringent than federal legislation. Local governments can pass laws specific to their communities (e.g., zoning restrictions), but they cannot pass legislation that weakens state laws.

LANGUAGE

English is the de facto national language, although Spanish is a widely used second language. Approximately 80% of the population speaks English, and 12% speaks Spanish as a first or second language. Chinese (Cantonese) is the third most common language spoken in the United States. In certain parts of the country (e.g., Louisiana, a former French colony), French, being the fourth most common language, is often commonly spoken. There are more than 300 languages spoken in the United States. In the western states, Korean, Chinese, Vietnamese, and Tagalog are frequently heard due to the immigration from the Asian countries to the West Coast.

RELIGION

In the United States, church and state have always been separate. In 2001, over three-quarters of the population considered themselves as Christian. About 13% of Americans identified themselves as non-religious or secular. Judaism accounted for about 1.4% of the population, whereas 0.6% of the population was Muslim, 0.5% was Buddhist, and 0.4% was Hindu. The major Christian denominations are Roman Catholic, Baptist, Methodist, Lutheran, Presbyterian, and Episcopalian.

TIME ZONES

The contiguous 48 states of United States have four time zones: Eastern, Central, Mountain, and Pacific, going from East to West. New York, on the east coast, is 5 hours behind Greenwich Mean Time (G.M.T.-5); California is 8 hours behind G.M.T. Alaska is 9 hours and Hawaii is 10 hours behind G.M.T.

BUSINESS PRACTICES

Punctuality is important. Generally in the United States the month is written first, then the date, then the year (e.g., January 16, 2007 or 1/16/2007). The work week is typically Monday through Friday, generally from 9 AM to 5 PM. Most offices will not be open on the weekends. Many convenience stores (those stores that sell frequently purchased products such as milk, snacks, bread) are open 24 hours.

Many people have business cards, but they are not exchanged unless there is a plan to contact the person at a later time. It is not mandatory to give a card in exchange for one received, and do not be offended if the person receiving a card places it in his/her back pocket; this is not a sign of disrespect!

TRAVEL

Americans tend to travel less to other countries than Europeans, who live in countries where borders are close to each other. In general, Americans are fascinated by people of other countries and are excited to meet them. Americans tend to have a poor sense of geography and enjoy speaking with international people about their country and traditions. The immense size of the United States allows Americans to travel great distances and see a wide variety of places that offer mountains, oceans, lakes, and large open areas without leaving the country.

FORMS OF ADDRESS

The order of most names is first name, middle name, and then last name. Always address a person with a title such as "Mr.," "Mrs.," "Ms.," "Dr.," or "Rev." with the last name only. As mentioned previously, if you are unclear as to whether a woman is married, refer to her as "Ms." It is appropriate to address a patient by their first name if they are under 18 years of age.

The letters "Jr." after a name stand for Junior and are sometimes found after a man's family name (e.g., John Smith, Jr.). This means that he was named after his father whose name was also John Smith. Another variation is the use of a Roman numeral after the name (e.g., John Smith III), meaning that he is the third generation with the same name as his predecessors. Both can be referred to as Mr. Smith.

FOOD

Food varies greatly in the United States and depends upon the region of the country and a family's heritage. People who have lived many generations in the United States tend to eat food common to the region in which they live (i.e., Tex-Mex, California cuisine, New England cuisine, Southern cuisine). Unfortunately, "American" cuisine has been often associated with the popular fast-food chains such as McDonald's, Burger King, Taco Bell, Wendy's, Pizza Hut, and Kentucky Fried Chicken. A fast-food restaurant is a **restaurant** characterized both by **food**, which is supplied quickly after ordering, and **service**, which is usually minimal. In a fast-food restaurant, you are expected to clear your own table.

Many fast-food restaurants have "drive-thru" windows to allow consumers to purchase fast food without having to park or exit their cars. Fortunately, these chains represent only a very small fraction of "American cuisine."

Lunch usually begins at 12:00 noon and ends around 2:00 PM. Americans do not take a "siesta" or break after the middle day meal. In fact, many business people do not close during the lunch hour at all. Dinner is the main meal for most people, starting between 5:30 and 8:00 PM. Proper eating etiquette calls for the fork to be held in the right hand. The knife is used for cutting, after the fork is either switched to the left hand or placed down on the table. After the food is cut, the fork is picked up again with the right hand.

It is not considered rude to eat while walking on the street, and many foods are eaten with the hands.

When eating out, the cost can be shared with friends. This is called "going Dutch" or "splitting the check."

GREETINGS

The usual greeting is a smile, often accompanied by a wave, nod, or handshake, and a verbal greeting. The handshake is very firm, but should not be painful! A weak handshake is often associated with weakness. Friends and family may greet each other with an embrace, but this is never done by a doctor with a patient on the first meeting. The greeting, "How are you?" is a general greeting and is usually not an inquiry about one's health except in the professional setting of a doctor meeting a patient.

GESTURES

In the United States, the average space between two parties is three feet. This distance may be closer or farther away from what is customary in other countries. In general, individuals of the same sex do not hold hands. If men hold hands, it is usually interpreted that they are "gay," having homosexual habits.

Gestures using your eyes, face, arms, hands, or legs are powerful forms of communication to punctuate even more than the spoken word. Unfortunately, these gestures do not have the same universal meanings. Gestures should be purposeful and reflective of the spoken word.

Facial gestures are important to understand. Because of the potential for misinterpretation, winking should not be used. It is inappropriate because of the flirtatious nature of the gesture. Sometimes a wink will indicate amusement and that the speaker is kidding. Shaking your head from side to side means "No," and shaking your head up and down means "Yes." It is impolite to pick your teeth, with or without a toothpick, in public.

To wave "goodbye" or say "hello" to someone, raise your hand and wave it from side to side, not front to back. You should wave the whole hand, not just the fingers. By waving the hand front to back or the fingers up and down, you are indicating "no", "stop", or "go away". By holding your hand up with the palm facing forward without movement means "stop".

To point, always use your index finger, although it is impolite to point at a person. Pointing with the middle finger or raising it alone will be interpreted as a rude gesture and is always to be avoided in the United States. Shaking a closed fist at someone is also rude, especially if it is in their face. This is an expression of anger.

To beckon someone in the United States, you should use all your fingers or just your index finger in a scooping motion with your palm facing upwards. Occasionally, the entire hand is flat with the palm up and the index finger or forefinger is wiggled to ask a person to come to you.

The "peace sign" or the "Victory sign" is shown by placing the palm out and the forefinger and index fingers are pointed upwards and split into the shape of a "V." The thumb crosses over the fourth finger. In some countries around the world, this has a rude meaning but not so in the United States.

Approval is often shown by the "OK sign" which is done by making a circle with the thumb and index finger. This means "all's well." Alternately, the "thumbs up" sign is done by making a fist and pointing the thumb straight upwards. Both of these signs for approval are acceptable gestures in the United States.

Although the sight of the soles of the shoe may be disrespectful in some cultures, it does not have any meaning in the United States. It is correct to sit with a leg crossed over the other knee in the United States.

Finally, when interviewing a patient, it is *not* rude to keep one or both of your hands in your pockets.

SMOKING, ALCOHOL, PRESCRIPTION MEDICATIONS, and RECREATIONAL DRUGS

Fewer and fewer public places (i.e., restaurants, hotels, office buildings) in the United States allow people to smoke cigarettes, cigars, or pipes. In some places, there are even anti-smoking laws. Alcohol is legal, but is restricted by age. The minimum drinking age is 21 in the United States. People need to show identification to verify their age in restaurants and in liquor stores.

There are sharp differences between prescription medications and illegal drugs. As mentioned earlier, when speaking to a patient always refer to illegal drugs (also known as illicit or street drugs) as recreational drugs! The United States has heavy penalties for the use and sale of recreational drugs such as marijuana, heroin, and cocaine, to name a few. Obviously, prescription medications may be also abused and used for purposes other than those indicated by the Food and Drug Administration (FDA).

SPORTS

The three most important spectator sports in the United States are baseball, football (American style), and basketball. Both the college and professional levels are popular. Major baseball teams play almost daily during the season, which lasts from April to October. The season culminates in the World Series. The football season begins in late summer and continues until midwinter. Other popular sports include ice hockey, auto racing, tennis, and soccer (known as football elsewhere in the world). Soccer tends to be more popular in the larger international cities of the United States where there are large immigrant populations. It is not nearly as popular as a professional sport in the United States as it is in other countries.

DRESS

The type of clothing worn is very much dependent upon the region of the country in which the person lives and works. Northeasterners tend to be more formal and wear more business dress, which consists of a shirt and tie for a man and a dress, blouse and skirt or slacks for a woman. Some people from Texas and the Southwest wear boots, large belt buckles, and cowboy hats. In the South, casual dress is more common than in the North. Of course, dress is often related to the climate. Northerners wear heavier clothes due to the colder weather. In cities, conservative business attire is the rule, whereas in rural areas clothing tends to be less formal.

EDUCATION

Education for children in the United States is compulsory. Most begin school around the age of 5. Some states allow children to leave school when they are 16 years of age; others require children to attend until age 18. Children age 5 attend kindergarten. Children ages 6–11 attend elementary or primary school (grades 1–5 or 6); children ages 11–14 attend middle or junior high school (grades 6 or 7–9 or 10); children ages 14–18 attend high school (grades 9 or 10–12). In the United States, there is both public and private education at all levels. Many, but not all, of the private institutions have religious affiliations. After high school, students can attend college. There are more than 1,500 universities and colleges in the United States. After college, students may elect to attend universities for higher educational degrees.

WORK

In large urban cities, many people use public transportation to get to work. However, most people in the United States commute to work by car. Full-time jobs are generally 37.5 hours per week. There is a minimum wage law requiring employers to pay a minimum wage for many employees. This wage can differ from state to state. Labor laws prohibit discrimination based on sex, age, race, religion, marital status, and political belief. Companies may offer health and dental insurance, as well as disability coverage. Often the most physically demanding jobs offer less compensation than those that are not physically demanding.

RELATIONSHIPS

Marriage laws are established by individual states. Marriages are presided by a minister, priest, rabbi, judge, Justice of the Peace, or other municipal officer. Only a few states allow same-sex marriages. Some states allow same-sex couples access to some benefits of marriage. Divorce laws vary from state to state.

BIRTHING

Most births in the United States occur in a hospital. The woman is placed in the lithotomy position for birthing. Many women believe that reliance on analgesic medication is unnatural, or worry that it may harm the child, but are still very concerned about labor pain. To alleviate pain, some women may undergo psychological preparation, education, massage, hypnosis, and water therapy. Most women also find helpful the emotional support and comfort measures by a husband, partner, or a trained professional. The Lamaze method of natural childbirth is very popular in the United States. Part of the Lamaze philosophy includes the understanding that women have the right to give birth free from routine medical interventions and that birth can safely take place in birth centers and homes.

Popular medical pain control for birthing in hospitals includes regional anesthetics, including **epidural** blocks, or **spinal anesthesia**. These anesthetics are a necessity for cesarean surgery, unless the patient undergoes surgery with a **general anesthetic**. Doctors in the United States often favor the epidural block because medication does not enter the mother's circulatory system, thus it does not cross the placenta and enter the bloodstream of the fetus.

Some women have midwives assist with their delivery instead of, or in addition to, an obstetrician. Midwives believe that childbirth is a normal process that is best accomplished with as little interference as possible. Midwives are trained to assist at births after having been certified.

DEATH

In some international cultures, the death of a loved one may be celebrated with music and festivities. In the United States, the death is usually more somber and accompanied with a time of mourning. Black is often worn to signify mourning. The deceased is usually embalmed and placed in a coffin for burial. Sometimes there is a viewing, where the deceased is displayed in the coffin in a chapel or funeral home for several days before the burial. Some religions (Jewish, for example) do not embalm the dead, who are buried generally within 24 hours of the death. No burials are performed on the Jewish Sabbath (Friday evening and Saturday). In the United States, there is no limit to the number of years that a body can remain in a cemetery. Cremation is an alternative to burial. In this procedure, the body is burned in a casket and the ashes can be buried, scattered over a site, or kept in an urn in the family's home.

HEALTH CARE

The United States government does not have universal health care or a system of socialized medicine. Patients without health care insurance must pay for service out of pocket (known as "fee-for-service") or be treated at another medical institution. Health care insurance is expensive and medical bills are extremely high. Health care insurance is generally, but not always, included as an employee benefit. Elderly, disabled, and poor individuals who are not covered by private insurance are covered by government insurance programs such as Medicare and Medicaid. As of 2001, 14.6% of the U.S. population, including 8.5 million children, had no health insurance coverage. A recent Harvard study showed that medical bills are the leading cause of bankruptcy in the United States.

Most health care in the United States occurs in the outpatient or "ambulatory care" setting generally in the form of clinics. There are also prenatal and family planning clinics, usually staffed by nurse practitioners. Home health care services are also available. For in-patient care there are for-profit hospitals and not-for-profit hospitals, generally run by the government, religious orders, or other not-for-profit organizations. Hospital emergency rooms care for emergencies but are also used frequently by patients for non-emergency care. In addition, hospice care is available for terminally ill patients who are expected to live six months or less.

HOLIDAYS

The United States Government recognizes ten federal holidays yearly. Many official holidays are celebrated on the Monday closest to the actual day of the holiday. The exceptions are New Year's Day, Thanksgiving, Christmas, Independence Day, and Veterans Day. Most retailers close on Thanksgiving and Christmas. The ten federal holidays and dates are:

January 1	New Year's Day
January, third Monday	Martin Luther King's Birthday
February, third Monday	George Washington's Birthday
May, last Monday	Memorial Day
July 4	Independence Day
September, first Monday	Labor Day
October, second Monday	Columbus Day
November 11	Veterans Day
November, fourth Thursday	Thanksgiving
December 25	Christmas Day

AMERICAN JARGON

Americans tend to use expressions that paint pictures, but the meaning of these figures of speech may be seen by others as a mix of strange words and be baffling. Take for example:

Ball park figure	Approximate value
Shotgun approach	Cover all areas
Raining cats and dogs	Raining extremely heavily

Rule of thumb	A rough guide; adequate working method
Down the tubes	Going bad
Flying by the seat of your pants	Doing something without proper training or instinct
Don't make waves	Don't cause trouble
Coming up roses	Going well
More than one way to skin a cat	More than one solution to a problem
Low ball	To offer an inappropriately low price to buy something
On a roll	Doing well
It will never fly	It will not work out
Run it up the flagpole	Check it out with superiors and get their advice

MISCELLANEOUS DO'S & DON'TS

Do use trash receptacles. Littering is frowned upon.
Do be respectful of police officers. Police officers expect to be addressed as "Sir," "Ma'am," or "Officer."
Do tip waiters, bartenders, and taxi drivers. Tips are not generally included in the cost of the service.
Do speak slowly and enunciate clearly, especially if you have an accent!
Do use gender neutral words instead of gender specific terms.

Don't wear jeans, jogging shoes, T-shirts, tight fitting sweaters (for women), tight fitting pants (for men) or hats when you are having any patient contact. Dress professionally!
Don't be overly physical when you greet someone.
Don't expect Americans to know much about your country.
Don't talk politics!
Don't use slang expressions or colloquialisms unless you fully understand the meaning.
Don't discuss religion
Don't use the term abortion. In the United States, "abortion" is an emotionally charged word. Instead ask a woman, "How many pregnancies have you had?" and "What was the outcome of the pregnancies?"

Finally, Americans can be sharply self-critical about the United States, but may take offense if they feel you are "bashing" America.

Section 4

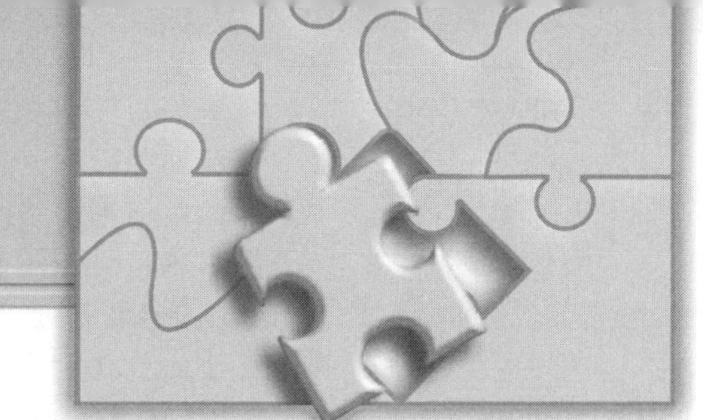

Practice Cases

General Case Instructions

This section consists of 30 practice cases[1] with more than 120 different diagnoses (see Appendix B). Each case has the following components:

- the **Examinee Instructions** (the information provided outside the room and duplicated in a folder in the room)
- the **Background Information** used for standardized patient (SP) training
- the **SP checklists** (history, physical examination, and interpersonal skills)
- a satisfactory **Patient Note**

You will note that the components of each case have different "voices":

- the voice of the director to the SP (Background Information)
- the voice of the SP to the candidate (History and Physical Exam Checklists)
- the voice of the candidate to another health care professional (Patient Note)

To maximize the usefulness of these cases, I suggest that you practice with a friend who has read the Background Information about the case and will play the role of the SP. The patient behavior, affect, and challenging questions are important in portraying the patient in the manner in which the case was written. Time yourself and record your interaction on an audiotape. After the 15-minute time period is up, listen to the tape and write down the questions that you asked.

[1]All cases are fictitious and names of the cases bear no relation to any persons alive or deceased.

Compare the questions you asked to the questions suggested for each case. Write up the Patient Note and compare it to the sample note included for each case. Differences in writing styles for the Patient Note are illustrated in different cases.

It is important to recognize that the history and physical examination checklists should not *be memorized!*

It is important to recognize that the history and physical examination checklists should *not* be memorized! They are only guides for the specific cases illustrated in this book.

The scores provided for each case area are to be used merely as a guide and bear no direct relation to the actual exam. The Spoken English Rating Scale is a scale from 1 to 5 with 3 being "average" and 5 being "excellent."

IMPORTANT NOTE: There is a major difference between interviewing an actual patient and an SP. In real life, one is instructed to ask many open-ended questions and allow the patient to answer each fully. On any SP-based assessment, the SPs are instructed *not* to provide any answers unless asked the question directly. Consequently, although a question such as, "*Do you have any other problems?*" may be a perfect question for real patients, an SP would answer, "*What do you mean?,*" requiring you to ask individual, direct questions as to whether the SP has, for example, chest pain, shortness of breath, nausea, vomiting, or diarrhea.

CASE 1—Ms. Martha Miller

Ms. Martha Miller, a 63-year-old woman, comes to clinic today complaining of recurrent headaches

VITAL SIGNS

Temperature: 98.6° F	**Pulse:** 80 regular
Blood Pressure: 135/75	**Respiratory Rate:** 12 regular

EXAMINEE'S TASKS

In the next 15 minutes, you are to:

1. Take a focused history
2. Do a focused physical examination
3. Discuss your initial clinical impressions and workup plans with the patient
4. Write the Patient Note after leaving the room

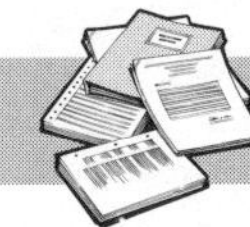

Examinee's Data Gathering (DG) Checklists

HISTORY CHECKLIST

1. ______
2. ______
3. ______
4. ______
5. ______
6. ______
7. ______
8. ______
9. ______
10. ______
11. ______
12. ______
13. ______
14. ______
15. ______
16. ______
17. ______
18. ______
19. ______
20. ______
21. ______

PHYSICAL EXAMINATION CHECKLIST

1. ______
2. ______
3. ______
4. ______
5. ______
6. ______
7. ______

8. ______________________________
9. ______________________________
10. ______________________________

Total DG Score ______ *Passing Score for DG is 22 points (70%)*

Examinee's Communication and Interpersonal Skills (CIS) Checklist

1. ______________________________
2. ______________________________
3. ______________________________
4. ______________________________
5. ______________________________
6. ______________________________
7. ______________________________
8. ______________________________
9. ______________________________
10. ______________________________
11. ______________________________
12. ______________________________
13. ______________________________
14. ______________________________
15. ______________________________
16. ______________________________
17. ______________________________
18. ______________________________
19. ______________________________
20. ______________________________

Total CIS Score ______ *Passing Score for CIS is 14 points (70%)*

123 Examinee's Spoken English Proficiency (SEP) Rating Scale

	Poor	Fair	Good	Very Good	Excellent
1. Ability of *patient* to understand *candidate*	1	2	3	4	5
2. Ability of *candidate* to understand *patient*	1	2	3	4	5
3. Candidate is articulate	1	2	3	4	5
4. Words are pronounced correctly	1	2	3	4	5
5. Range of vocabulary and sentence structure	1	2	3	4	5
6. Stress, rhythm, and intonation	1	2	3	4	5
7. Grammar	1	2	3	4	5
8. Repair strategies	1	2	3	4	5

Total SEP Score ______ *Passing Score for SEP is 28 points (70%)*

Examinee's Patient Note (PN)

HISTORY—Include any significant pertinent positives and negatives from the history

PHYSICAL EXAMINATION—Include any significant pertinent positives and negatives

DIFFERENTIAL DIAGNOSIS

In order of likelihood, write no more than five (5) differential diagnoses

1.
2.
3.
4.
5.

DIAGNOSTIC WORKUP

Immediate plans, write no more than five (5) diagnostic studies

1.
2.
3.
4.
5.

Alleviating a patient's overwhelming worry can go a long way toward calming them, and, ultimately helping them. This kind of patient care is often neglected, and is very important.

Background Information for Standardized Patient

PATIENT BEHAVIOR

Occasionally rubs her hands over her right eye

AFFECT

In pain, not happy

PROVOCATIVE QUESTION(S) AND PLAUSIBLE ANSWER(S)

"Could this be a brain tumor like my sister?" "The pain is so bad; will anything help me?"

"I am glad you came in. I certainly can't tell at this point exactly what is causing your pain, but we will do our absolute best to figure it out, and to get you the proper pain mediation."

CHIEF COMPLAINT

"Recurrent headaches"

HISTORY OF PRESENT ILLNESS

Martha Miller is a 63-year-old retired college English teacher who is complaining of recurrent headaches for the past 4–5 months. She has a history of migraine headaches for over 20 years. They were always relieved by taking two Fiorinal tablets every 4–6 hours. The migraines would last 6–8 hours and would occur about once a month. Now for the past 4–5 months she has been getting 2–3 headaches a day, and they are only partially relieved by the Fiorinal. The headaches are pressurelike sensations over the right eye with gradual onset and move down the back of the neck. They are about an 8 on a 10-point scale. The headaches seem to improve with rest and closing the eyes. She doesn't think anything really precipitates the headaches. There is no history of head injury, nausea, vomiting, eye pain on exposure to light, fever, weakness, "pins and needles" sensation, dizziness, or visual disturbances. There are no changes in mental status, confusion, or difficulty in speech.

PAST MEDICAL HISTORY

She's been healthy all her life. The only surgery was a tonsillectomy as a child.

MEDICATIONS

Fiorinal for headaches

ALLERGIES

None

SOCIAL HISTORY
There is no history of recreational drug use. She drinks wine on weekends socially with friends. She used to smoke about 2 packs per day for about 20 years, but stopped about 5 years ago.

FAMILY HISTORY
She is married to Alex for the past 38 years. They have one son, Jeremy, age 33 years, who is single. About 6 months ago, she learned that her son is gay and is terribly upset by that situation. Martha and Alex live in a home in the suburban Northwest. Her husband, an architect, sold his firm and retired about 6 months ago. Unfortunately, he has no hobbies and just sits at home watching television. Martha's younger sister Claire died 2 years ago of a brain tumor, and Martha is concerned that she also may have one. Claire also had headaches. An older brother, a cigarette smoker, died of lung cancer at age 67 years about 5 years ago.

SEXUAL HISTORY
She is monogamous with husband only and has sex about once or twice a month.

REVIEW OF SYSTEMS
Noncontributory

SP's Data Gathering (DG) Checklists

HISTORY CHECKLIST

1. I am a retired college English teacher.
2. I have a history of migraines for the past 20 years.
3. The migraines would last 6–8 hours.
4. The migraines were relieved by taking 2 Fiorinal tablets every 4–6 hours.
5. I would get the migraines about once a month.
6. For the past 4–5 months, I have been getting 2–3 headaches a day.
7. They are relieved by rest and closing the eyes and are only partially relieved by Fiorinal.
8. The headaches are pressurelike sensations over the right eye with gradual onset and down the back of the neck.
9. They are about an 8 on a 10-point scale.
10. I don't know of anything that precipitates the headaches.
11. There is no history of head trauma.
12. There is no history of nausea or vomiting.
13. There is no history of preceding aura, eye pain on exposure to light, fever, weakness, "pins and needles" sensation, dizziness, or visual disturbances (any two).
14. There are no changes in mental status; I am not confused; I do not have difficulty in speech (any one).
15. I have no allergies.
16. I drink wine socially with friends.
17. About 6 months ago, I learned that my son Jeremy is gay.
18. I am terribly upset that my son is gay.
19. My husband Alex retired 6 months ago.
20. My younger sister Claire died 2 years ago of a brain tumor.
21. I am worried that I have a brain tumor.

PHYSICAL CHECKLIST

1. Evaluated pupillary reflexes
2. Performed an ophthalmoscopic examination in both eyes
3. Palpated sinuses
4. Evaluated neck for rigidity
5. Evaluated cranial nerves III, IV, and VI (EOMs)
6. Evaluated for gross sensory deficits
7. Evaluated for gross motor deficits
8. Tested deep tendon reflexes (at least 1 in upper and 1 in lower extremity)
9. Tested muscle strength
10. Checked for tenderness over temporal artery

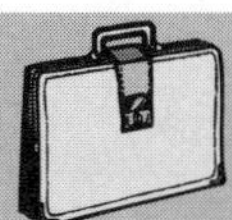

SP's Communication and Interpersonal Skills (CIS) Checklist

1. Knocked before entering
2. Opened interview by introducing self
3. Addressed patient using last name with introduction (e.g., Ms. Miller)
4. Appearance (e.g., clean and neat)
5. Allowed patient to express reason for seeking medical attention
6. Made comfortable eye contact
7. Did *not* use leading/biased questions (e.g., "You don't have..." or "You're not...")
8. Asked questions individually
9. Did *not* use the "Why" question
10. Concentrated and focused on patient's needs
11. Maintained comfortable and appropriate distance
12. Gave patient time to think and answer without interrupting
13. Used proper draping during physical exam
14. Did physical examination in an orderly manner
15. Summarized patient's condition (or asked patient to summarize)
16. Discussed diagnostic tests and/or next step in treatment in lay terms
17. Asked whether patient had other questions/concerns
18. Provided patient education/suggestions where appropriate
19. Did *not* give false assurances
20. Showed empathy

123 SP's Spoken English Proficiency (SEP) Rating Scale

	Poor	Fair	Good	Very Good	Excellent
1. Ability of *patient* to understand *candidate*	1	2	3	4	5
2. Ability of *candidate* to understand *patient*	1	2	3	4	5
3. Candidate is articulate	1	2	3	4	5
4. Words are pronounced correctly	1	2	3	4	5
5. Range of vocabulary and sentence structure	1	2	3	4	5
6. Stress, rhythm, and intonation	1	2	3	4	5
7. Grammar	1	2	3	4	5
8. Repair strategies	1	2	3	4	5

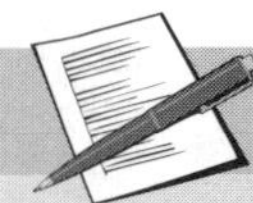

Example of a Satisfactory Patient Note (PN)

HISTORY—Include any significant pertinent positives and negatives

Ms. Martha Miller is a 63-year-old retired college English teacher who is complaining of recurrent headaches for the past 4–5 months. The patient has a 20-year history of migraine headaches. She presents today for a change in the pattern of her headaches. The migraines, which she would get about once a month, were relieved by taking 2 Fiorinal tablets every 4–6 hours. For the past 4–5 months, she has been experiencing 2–3 headaches a day unrelieved by the Fiorinal. She describes them as pressurelike sensations over the right eye with gradual onset and down the back of the neck. They are about an 8 on a 10-point scale. The headaches seem to improve with rest and closing the eyes. She is unaware of any precipitating factor. There is no history of head trauma, nausea, vomiting, photophobia, fever, weakness, paresthesia, dizziness, or visual disturbances. There is no change in mental status, no confusion, and no difficulty in speech.

About 6 months ago, she learned that her son is gay, and she is terribly upset about it. Her husband recently retired and sits at home all day. In addition, she is concerned that she may have a brain tumor as her younger sister died 2 years ago of a brain tumor, and her sister also had headaches.

The patient enjoys drinking wine with friends on weekends; there is no other recreational drug use. She has no known allergy.

PHYSICAL EXAMINATION—Include any significant pertinent positives and negatives

Physical examination reveals a well-developed, well-nourished, 63-year-old woman, appearing somewhat older than her stated age, complaining of a right-sided headache. Vital signs are normal. Pupillary reflexes are normal. Ophthalmoscopic examination reveals normal discs and vasculature. There is no tenderness over the frontal, ethmoid, or maxillary sinuses. There is no nuchal rigidity. Cranial nerves II–XII are intact. Gross sensory and motor nerves are normal. The DTRs (biceps, triceps, patella, and Achilles) are normal and equal bilaterally. Muscle strength is 2+ bilaterally in the upper and lower extremities. There is no tenderness or swelling over the temporal arteries.

DIFFERENTIAL DIAGNOSIS

In order of likelihood, write no more than five (5) differential diagnoses

1. Migraine headache
2. Tension headache
3. R/O brain tumor
4. R/O temporal arteritis
5. Depression

DIAGNOSTIC WORKUP

Immediate plans, write no more than five (5) diagnostic studies

1. CBC, ESR
2. Lumbar puncture
3. CT scan of the head and sinuses
4. Temporal artery biopsy
5. ____________________

CASE 2—Ms. Peggy Graham

Ms. Peggy Graham, a 45-year-old woman, presents to clinic complaining of abdominal pain.

VITAL SIGNS

Temperature: 99.4° F	**Pulse:** 90 regular
Blood Pressure: 135/80	**Respiratory Rate:** 14 regular

EXAMINEE'S TASKS

In the next 15 minutes, you are to:

1) Take a focused history
2) Do a focused physical examination
3) Discuss your initial clinical impressions and workup plans with the patient
4) Write the Patient Note after leaving the room

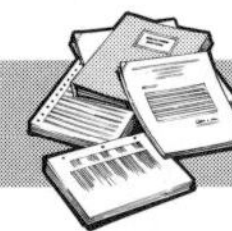

Examinee's Data Gathering (DG) Checklists

HISTORY CHECKLIST

1. ______
2. ______
3. ______
4. ______
5. ______
6. ______
7. ______
8. ______
9. ______
10. ______
11. ______
12. ______
13. ______
14. ______
15. ______
16. ______
17. ______
18. ______
19. ______
20. ______
21. ______
22. ______

PHYSICAL EXAMINATION CHECKLIST

1. ______
2. ______
3. ______
4. ______
5. ______

6. ______________________________
7. ______________________________

Total DG Score ______ *Passing Score for DG is 20 points (70%)*

Examinee's Communication and Interpersonal Skills (CIS) Checklist

1. ______________________________
2. ______________________________
3. ______________________________
4. ______________________________
5. ______________________________
6. ______________________________
7. ______________________________
8. ______________________________
9. ______________________________
10. ______________________________
11. ______________________________
12. ______________________________
13. ______________________________
14. ______________________________
15. ______________________________
16. ______________________________
17. ______________________________
18. ______________________________
19. ______________________________
20. ______________________________

Total CIS Score ______ *Passing Score for CIS is 14 points (70%)*

123 Examinee's Spoken English Proficiency (SEP) Rating Scale

	Poor	Fair	Good	Very Good	Excellent
1. Ability of *patient* to understand *candidate*	1	2	3	4	5
2. Ability of *candidate* to understand *patient*	1	2	3	4	5
3. Candidate is articulate	1	2	3	4	5
4. Words are pronounced correctly	1	2	3	4	5
5. Range of vocabulary and sentence structure	1	2	3	4	5
6. Stress, rhythm, and intonation	1	2	3	4	5
7. Grammar	1	2	3	4	5
8. Repair strategies	1	2	3	4	5

Total SEP Score _____ *Passing Score for SEP is 28 points (70%)*

Examinee's Patient Note (PN)

HISTORY—Include any significant pertinent positives and negatives from the history

PHYSICAL EXAMINATION—Include any significant pertinent positives and negatives

DIFFERENTIAL DIAGNOSIS

In order of likelihood, write no more than five (5) differential diagnoses

1.
2.
3.
4.
5.

DIAGNOSTIC WORKUP

Immediate plans, write no more than five (5) diagnostic studies

1.
2.
3.
4.
5.

Background Information for Standardized Patient

PATIENT BEHAVIOR

Tends to use one-word answers; cuts the doctor off at times when answering questions; doesn't want to be here

AFFECT

Curt, dismissive of the doctor; doesn't trust doctors

PROVOCATIVE QUESTION(S) AND PLAUSIBLE ANSWER(S)

"Look, what the hell is wrong with me, and can you give me something to make the pain go away?"

"I am sorry for your pain, and just as soon as I have asked you some questions and done a physical exam, I will do my best to get you the proper treatment for your pain."

Remember that a patient may not readily admit the actual amount of alcohol they consume. Watch for body language and any hesitations, or change in voice or posture, when someone is answering these questions.

CHIEF COMPLAINT

"My stomach hurts a lot"

HISTORY OF PRESENT ILLNESS

Peggy Graham is a 45-year-old, slightly obese housewife who presents to the clinic with abdominal pain. The pain is located in the upper center and in the right upper quadrant of her abdomen. The pain started about 10 days ago. It seems to come and go. At worst, it is about an 8 out of 10. It seems to be getting worse, which is why she came in today for evaluation. The pain often goes straight through to her back but sometimes up to her right shoulder. It's burning or gnawing in nature. She has noticed that food, antacids, cimetidine, and Pepto-Bismol make it better, but heavy meals and fatty foods seem to make it worse. The pain tends to get better for about 2–3 hours after she eats a nonfatty meal, and then slowly gets progressively worse again.

Over the past 10 days, she has felt nauseated several times, but only vomited this morning. The vomit was yellow in color and was very sour tasting. There was no blood in the vomit. There has been no diarrhea or constipation. There is no blood in the stools. The stools are normal in color. There has been no weight loss. She has never had this type of pain before.

PAST MEDICAL HISTORY

She has been very healthy all her life. There is no history of surgery.

MEDICATIONS
Cimetidine, Pepto-Bismol, and antacids for recent problem; aspirin when she has a shoulder ache.

ALLERGIES
None

FAMILY HISTORY
She has been married for 18 years and has three children: a son age 16 years, a daughter age 14 years, and another daughter age 11 years. All children live at home with her and her husband.

SOCIAL HISTORY
She admits to drinking about 2 glasses of wine about three times a week. In the past month, she has suspected that her husband has been having an affair with a friend's wife. Her alcoholic consumption has increased to a few shots a day. She has never smoked or used other recreational drugs.

SEXUAL HISTORY
She is monogamous with only her husband and had sex normally about 1–2 times a week until about a month ago. Since then, she has had no sexual relations.

REVIEW OF SYSTEMS
Noncontributory

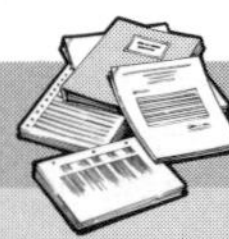

SP's Data Gathering (DG) Checklists

HISTORY CHECKLIST

1. I am a housewife.
2. I live at home with my husband and three children
3. The abdominal pain started about 10 days ago.
4. The pain is located in the upper center and right upper part of my abdomen.
4. The pain seems to come and go.
5. At worst, the pain is about an 8 out of 10.
6. The pain often goes straight through to my back, but sometimes up to my right shoulder blade.
7. The pain is burning or gnawing in nature.
8. Food, antacids, cimetidine, and Pepto-Bismol make it better.
9. Heavy meals and fatty foods make it worse.
10. I have felt nauseated several times in the past 10 days.
11. I vomited once this morning.
12. The vomit was yellow in color and was very sour tasting.
13. There was no blood in the vomit.
14. I have not had diarrhea or constipation.
15. There is no blood in the stools.
16. I have had no weight loss.
17. I have never had surgery.
18. I drink about 2 glasses of wine about three times a week.
19. I have increased my alcoholic consumption to a few shots a day over the past 8–10 days.
20. I take aspirin when I have a shoulder ache.
21. I never have smoked.
22. I have no allergies.

PHYSICAL CHECKLIST

1. Took blood pressure
2. Evaluated for orthostatic hypotension
3. Performed light palpation of the abdomen in all 4 quadrants *after* auscultation
4. Performed deep palpation of the abdomen in all 4 quadrants
5. Elicited for rebound abdominal tenderness
6. Percussed abdomen in all 4 quadrants
7. Evaluated liver by palpation

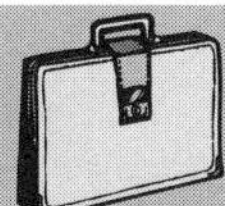

SP's Communication and Interpersonal Skills (CIS) Checklist

1. Knocked before entering
2. Opened interview by introducing self
3. Addressed patient using last name with introduction (e.g., Ms. Graham)
4. Appearance (e.g., clean and neat)
5. Allowed patient to express reason for seeking medical attention
6. Made comfortable eye contact
7. Did *not* use leading/biased questions (e.g., "You don't have…" or "You're not…")
8. Asked questions individually
9. Did *not* use the "Why" question
10. Concentrated and focused on patient's needs
11. Maintained comfortable and appropriate distance
12. Gave patient time to think and answer without interrupting
13. Used proper draping during physical exam
14. Did physical examination in an orderly manner
15. Summarized patient's condition (or asked patient to summarize)
16. Discussed diagnostic tests and/or next step in treatment in lay terms
17. Asked whether patient had other questions/concerns
18. Provided patient education/suggestions where appropriate
19. Did *not* give false reassurances
20. Showed empathy

123 SP's Spoken English Proficiency (SEP) Rating Scale

	Poor	Fair	Good	Very Good	Excellent
1. Ability of *patient* to understand *candidate*	1	2	3	4	5
2. Ability of *candidate* to understand *patient*	1	2	3	4	5
3. Candidate is articulate	1	2	3	4	5
4. Words are pronounced correctly	1	2	3	4	5
5. Range of vocabulary and sentence structure	1	2	3	4	5
6. Stress, rhythm, and intonation	1	2	3	4	5
7. Grammar	1	2	3	4	5
8. Repair strategies	1	2	3	4	5

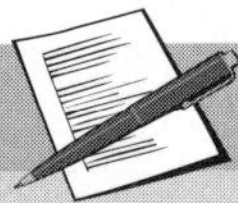

Example of a Satisfactory Patient Note (PN)

HISTORY—Include any significant pertinent positives and negatives

Ms. Peggy Graham is a 45-year-old, slightly obese housewife, mother of three children, who presents to the clinic with abdominal pain for the past 10 days that has been getting worse. The pain is located in the epigastrium and in the right upper quadrant of her abdomen. The pain seems to come and go; at its worst, it is about an 8 out of 10. The patient describes the pain as burning or gnawing, that often goes straight through to her back but sometimes up to her right shoulder. She has noticed that food, antacids, cimetidine, and Pepto-Bismol make it better, but heavy meals and fatty foods seem to make it worse. The pain tends to get better for about 2–3 hours after she eats a nonfatty meal, and then slowly gets progressively worse again. Over the past 10 days, she has felt nauseated several times, but vomited only this morning. The vomit was yellow in color and was very sour tasting. There was no blood in the vomit. There has been no diarrhea or constipation. There is no blood in the stools. The stools are normal in color. There has been no weight loss. She has never had this type of pain before. She takes no medications except aspirin when she has a shoulder ache. There is no history of surgery.

The patient admits to drinking about 2 glasses of wine about three times a week. Recently, she has suspected her husband of having an affair with a friend's wife. Her alcoholic consumption has increased to a few shots a day. She has never smoked or used recreational drugs other than alcohol. She has no known allergy.

PHYSICAL EXAMINATION—Include any significant pertinent positives and negatives

Physical examination reveals a well-developed, slightly obese, 45-year-old woman, appearing her stated age, complaining of right upper quadrant abdominal pain. Vital signs are normal; there is no change in BP with postural changes. The abdomen is slightly distended. Bowel sounds are present. There is mild tenderness in the right upper quadrant. Murphy's sign is present. No masses are palpated. The liver span is 10 cm in the midclavicular line.

DIFFERENTIAL DIAGNOSIS

In order of likelihood, write no more than five (5) differential diagnoses

1. Cholecystitis
2. R/O pancreatitis
3. R/O peptic ulcer disease
4. R/O GERD
5. R/O gastritis

DIAGNOSTIC WORKUP

Immediate plans, write no more than five (5) diagnostic studies

1. Rectal exam and stool for FOBT
2. CBC, amylase, lipase, AST, ALT
3. HIDA scan
4. Upper GI endoscopy
5. Upper barium GI study

CASE 3—Mr. Philip Ross

Mr. Philip Ross, a 35-year-old man, presents to clinic complaining of lower back pain.

VITAL SIGNS

Temperature: 98.4° F	**Pulse:** 85 regular
Blood Pressure: 125/75	**Respiratory Rate:** 12 regular

EXAMINEE'S TASKS

In the next 15 minutes, you are to:

1) Take a focused history
2) Do a focused physical examination
3) Discuss your initial clinical impressions and workup plans with the patient
4) Write the Patient Note after leaving the room

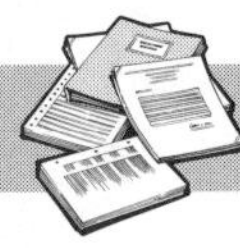

Examinee's Data Gathering (DG) Checklists

HISTORY CHECKLIST

1. __________
2. __________
3. __________
4. __________
5. __________
6. __________
7. __________
8. __________
9. __________
10. __________
11. __________
12. __________
13. __________
14. __________
15. __________
16. __________
17. __________
18. __________
19. __________
20. __________

PHYSICAL EXAMINATION CHECKLIST

1. __________
2. __________
3. __________
4. __________
5. __________
6. __________
7. __________

8. ______________________________

Total DG Score _____ *Passing Score for DG is 20 points (70%)*

Examinee's Communication and Interpersonal Skills (CIS) Checklist

1. ______________________________
2. ______________________________
3. ______________________________
4. ______________________________
5. ______________________________
6. ______________________________
7. ______________________________
8. ______________________________
9. ______________________________
10. ______________________________
11. ______________________________
12. ______________________________
13. ______________________________
14. ______________________________
15. ______________________________
16. ______________________________
17. ______________________________
18. ______________________________
19. ______________________________
20. ______________________________

Total CIS Score _____ *Passing Score for CIS is 14 points (70%)*

123 Examinee's Spoken English Proficiency (SEP) Rating Scale

	Poor	Fair	Good	Very Good	Excellent
1. Ability of *patient* to understand *candidate*	1	2	3	4	5
2. Ability of *candidate* to understand *patient*	1	2	3	4	5
3. Candidate is articulate	1	2	3	4	5
4. Words are pronounced correctly	1	2	3	4	5
5. Range of vocabulary and sentence structure	1	2	3	4	5
6. Stress, rhythm, and intonation	1	2	3	4	5
7. Grammar	1	2	3	4	5
8. Repair strategies	1	2	3	4	5

Total SEP Score ______ *Passing Score for SEP is 28 points (70%)*

Examinee's Patient Note (PN)

HISTORY—Include any significant pertinent positives and negatives

PHYSICAL EXAMINATION—Include any significant pertinent positives and negatives

DIFFERENTIAL DIAGNOSIS

In order of likelihood, write no more than five (5) differential diagnoses

1.
2.
3.
4.
5.

DIAGNOSTIC WORKUP

Immediate plans, write no more than five (5) diagnostic studies

1.
2.
3.
4.
5.

Background Information for Standardized Patient

PATIENT BEHAVIOR

Lying down, not moving around much; answers questions readily

AFFECT

In a great deal of pain

PROVOCATIVE QUESTION(S) AND PLAUSIBLE ANSWER(S)

"Doc, can you just give me something to make this go away? I can't even think straight!"

"I can see you are in a great deal of pain, and I will complete the exam as quickly as I can. As soon as I do, we will hopefully be able to see what is wrong, and get you the proper treatment."

A helpful question for almost all cases is to ask, "How is this affecting your everyday life?"

CHIEF COMPLAINT

"I've got lower back pain and it's killing me."

HISTORY OF PRESENT ILLNESS

Philip Ross is a 35-year-old who presents to clinic for evaluation of lower back pain. He states that the pain began about 4 days ago after he helped his friend move. He picked up a mattress and felt his back go into spasm. The pain is aching and is very deep in his lower back, worse on the left side above his hip. He denies any pain shooting down his legs. The pain is about an 8 out of 10. Lying flat in bed makes it better. When he tries to twist his waist, it hurts the most. He has also noticed that sitting for more than 15 minutes and walking makes it hurt more. He has had to miss work for the last day and a half as the pain has been too great. He bought some ibuprofen 400 mg, and he takes it about every 6–8 hours; it makes the pain more tolerable. There is no urinary or fecal incontinence. There are no night sweats or fever associated with the pain. There is no numbness in his feet. He has had a history of occasional back pain usually when he walks too much.

PAST MEDICAL HISTORY

He has been in good health except for the back pain. He had an appendectomy at age 23.

MEDICATIONS

None except the ibuprofen.

ALLERGIES

None

SOCIAL HISTORY

He is a high school math teacher. He was married for 10 years but has been divorced for 2 years. He has a 7-year-old daughter who lives with his ex-wife. He sees her about once or twice a month. He is a one-pack-per-day cigarette smoker for about 15 years. He drinks beer, about a six-pack every weekend.

FAMILY HISTORY

His mother is 55 years old and is in good health; father is 57 years old and has diabetes. He has a brother age 32 years whom he doesn't see often as he lives far away.

SEXUAL HISTORY

He lives with his girlfriend of 1 year in an apartment house. They have sex 4–5 times a week. There is no other sexual partner.

REVIEW OF SYSTEMS

Noncontributory

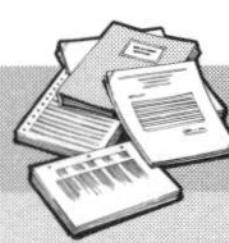

SP's Data Gathering (DG) Checklists

HISTORY CHECKLIST

1. I have bad back pain.
2. The pain started 4 days ago.
3. I was helping a friend move a mattress when it started.
4. The pain is aching and is very deep in my lower back.
5. It is worse on my left side above my hip.
6. I do not have any pain shooting down my legs.
7. The pain is about an 8 out of 10.
8. I find that lying flat in bed makes it better.
9. When I try to twist at my waist, it hurts the most.
10. It also hurts when I sit for more than 15 minutes or walk.
11. I have missed a day and a half of work because of the pain.
12. I take ibuprofen 400 mg about every 6–8 hours for the pain.
13. The ibuprofen makes the pain more tolerable.
14. I do not have any urinary incontinence.
15. I do not have any fecal incontinence.
16. I do not have night sweats or fever associated with the pain.
17. There is no numbness in my feet.
18. I have a history of occasional back pain usually when I walk too much.
19. I have no allergies.
20. I am a high school math teacher.

PHYSICAL CHECKLIST

1. Palpated lower back
2. Evaluated range of motion by having patient flex, extend, tilt laterally and rotate torso at waist (3 of 4 required)
3. Performed straight leg raising
4. Assessed deep tendon reflexes (patella and Achilles)
5. Assessed sensation in lower extremities
6. Assessed muscle strength in lower extremities
7. Assessed gait
8. Palpated abdomen

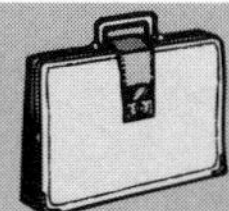

SP's Communication and Interpersonal Skills (CIS) Checklist

1. Knocked before entering
2. Opened interview by introducing self
3. Addressed patient using last name with introduction (e.g., Mr. Roth)
4. Appearance (e.g., clean and neat)
5. Allowed patient to express reason for seeking medical attention
6. Made comfortable eye contact
7. Did *not* use leading/biased questions (e.g., "You don't have..." or "You're not...")
8. Asked questions individually
9. Did *not* use the "Why" question
10. Concentrated and focused on patient's needs
11. Maintained comfortable and appropriate distance
12. Gave patient time to think and answer without interrupting
13. Used proper draping during physical exam
14. Did physical examination in an orderly manner
15. Summarized patient's condition (or asked patient to summarize)
16. Discussed diagnostic tests and/or next step in treatment in lay terms
17. Asked whether patient had other questions/concerns
18. Provided patient education/suggestions where appropriate
19. Did *not* give false assurances
20. Showed empathy

123 SP's Spoken English Proficiency (SEP) Rating Scale

	Poor	Fair	Good	Very Good	Excellent
1. Ability of *patient* to understand *candidate*	1	2	3	4	5
2. Ability of *candidate* to understand *patient*	1	2	3	4	5
3. Candidate is articulate	1	2	3	4	5
4. Words are pronounced correctly	1	2	3	4	5
5. Range of vocabulary and sentence structure	1	2	3	4	5
6. Stress, rhythm, and intonation	1	2	3	4	5
7. Grammar	1	2	3	4	5
8. Repair strategies	1	2	3	4	5

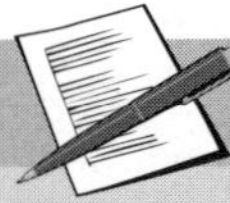

Example of a Satisfactory Patient Note (PN)

HISTORY—Include any significant pertinent positives and negatives

Mr. Philip Roth is a 35-year-old high school math teacher whose chief complaint is "I've got lower back pain and it's killing me. Give me some pain meds!" The pain started about 4 days ago when he was helping his friend move a mattress. He felt his back immediately go into spasm. The patient describes the pain as aching and very deep in his lower back. It is worse on the left side above his hip. He denies any pain shooting down his legs. The pain is about an 8 out of 10. Lying flat in bed makes it better. When he tries to twist his waist, it hurts the most. He has also noticed that sitting for more than 15 minutes and walking makes it hurt more. He takes ibuprofen 400 mg about every 6–8 hours, which makes the pain more tolerable. The patient denies any urinary or fecal incontinence. There is no history of night sweats or fever. The patient does not describe numbness in his feet. He does describe having had occasional back pain when he walks too much.

PHYSICAL EXAMINATION—Include any significant pertinent positives and negatives

Physical examination reveals a well-developed, well-nourished 35-year-old man appearing his stated age, lying on the exam table and complaining of lower back pain. Vital signs are within normal limits. Palpation of abdomen reveals no abnormalities. Palpation of the lower back reveals generalized tenderness. The patient is unable to be evaluated for range of motion because of the pain. A straight-leg raising test is positive when the left leg is raised about 45 degrees. DTRs are within normal limits. Gross sensory and motor responses are within normal limits. Evaluation of gait shows slight favoring of the left leg. No footdrop is detected.

DIFFERENTIAL DIAGNOSIS

In order of likelihood, write no more than five (5) differential diagnoses

1. Lumbar muscular strain
2. R/O acute disc herniation
3. R/O lumbar spinal stenosis
4. R/O degenerative arthritis
5. R/O malignancy

DIAGNOSTIC WORKUP

Immediate plans, write no more than five (5) diagnostic studies

1. X-ray of lumbar spine
2. CBC, calcium, BUN, creatinine
3. MRI of lumbar spine
4. SPEP, PSA
5. Rectal exam and stool for FOBT

CASE 4—Ms. Judy Manoff

Ms. Judy Manoff, a 51-year-old woman, presents to clinic complaining of left wrist pain and loss of sensation in her left fingers.

VITAL SIGNS

Temperature: 98.6° F	**Pulse:** 70 regular
Blood Pressure: 130/80	**Respiratory Rate:** 10 regular

EXAMINEE'S TASKS

In the next 15 minutes, you are to:

1) Take a focused history
2) Do a focused physical examination
3) Discuss your initial clinical impressions and workup plans with the patient
4) Write the Patient Note after leaving the room

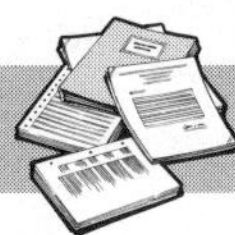

Examinee's Data Gathering (DG) Checklists

HISTORY CHECKLIST

1. ____________________
2. ____________________
3. ____________________
4. ____________________
5. ____________________
6. ____________________
7. ____________________
8. ____________________
9. ____________________
10. ____________________
11. ____________________
12. ____________________
13. ____________________
14. ____________________
15. ____________________
16. ____________________
17. ____________________
18. ____________________
19. ____________________
20. ____________________
21. ____________________

PHYSICAL EXAMINATION CHECKLIST

1. ____________________
2. ____________________
3. ____________________
4. ____________________
5. ____________________
6. ____________________

Total DG Score ______ *Passing Score for DG is 19 points (70%)*

Examinee's Communication and Interpersonal Skills (CIS) Checklist

1. ______________________________
2. ______________________________
3. ______________________________
4. ______________________________
5. ______________________________
6. ______________________________
7. ______________________________
8. ______________________________
9. ______________________________
10. ______________________________
11. ______________________________
12. ______________________________
13. ______________________________
14. ______________________________
15. ______________________________
16. ______________________________
17. ______________________________
18. ______________________________
19. ______________________________
20. ______________________________

Total CIS Score ______ *Passing Score for CIS is 14 points (70%)*

123 Examinee's Spoken English Proficiency (SEP) Rating Scale

	Poor	Fair	Good	Very Good	Excellent
1. Ability of *patient* to understand *candidate*	1	2	3	4	5
2. Ability of *candidate* to understand *patient*	1	2	3	4	5
3. Candidate is articulate	1	2	3	4	5
4. Words are pronounced correctly	1	2	3	4	5
5. Range of vocabulary and sentence structure	1	2	3	4	5
6. Stress, rhythm, and intonation	1	2	3	4	5
7. Grammar	1	2	3	4	5
8. Repair strategies	1	2	3	4	5

Total SEP Score ______ *Passing Score for SEP is 28 points (70%)*

Examinee's Patient Note (PN)

HISTORY—Include any significant pertinent positives and negatives

PHYSICAL EXAMINATION— Include any significant pertinent positives and negatives

DIFFERENTIAL DIAGNOSIS

In order of likelihood, write no more than five (5) differential diagnoses

1.
2.
3.
4.
5.

DIAGNOSTIC WORKUP

Immediate plans, write no more than five (5) diagnostic studies

1.
2.
3.
4.
5.

Background Information for Standardized Patient

PATIENT BEHAVIOR
Unremarkable

AFFECT
Concerned, nice patient

PROVOCATIVE QUESTION(S) AND PLAUSIBLE ANSWER(S)
"Could this be an early sign of having a stroke?"

"It is highly unlikely that this could be a stroke, but let's get some tests first."

CHIEF COMPLAINT
"Numbness and pain in my left wrist and fingers"

HISTORY OF PRESENT ILLNESS
Judy Manoff is a 51-year-old woman who presents to clinic for evaluation of wrist pain. She is employed as a secretary and for the last 3 weeks has noticed pain in her left wrist and numbness and burning in the ring and pinky fingers on her left hand. The pain seems to be getting worse. She describes that she also has a sensory loss in the same fingers. Over the past week, she has noted inability to use her left hand to button or unbutton her clothing. She is extremely upset about her symptoms because she is right handed and uses the computer mouse with her right hand only. She is wondering why this is occurring in the hand she doesn't use as much. She is concerned that she might be having a stroke like her mother had several years ago. There is no tingling in the left arm or neck. She is unaware of anything that makes it better or worse. There is no difficulty in speech or in vision.

PAST MEDICAL HISTORY
She has been in good health except for mild hypertension and high cholesterol, both well controlled with medications. There is no history of rheumatoid arthritis, diabetes, or thyroid disease.

MEDICATIONS
Atenolol 50 mg daily for hypertension
Lipitor 20 mg daily for high cholesterol

ALLERGIES
Shellfish (rash)

A patient's hobbies and interests are not always just "small talk." They sometimes have a direct impact on the patient's present condition. At minimum, this information will help establish rapport; at maximum it will directly affect your diagnosis.

SOCIAL HISTORY

She is happily married for the past 27 years. She has two children: Brian, age 25; and Margaret, age 22. She lives with her husband, who is an attorney, in rural, upper New York State. She denies any alcohol or other recreational drug use. She did try marijuana in college. She is very athletic and enjoys yoga and mountain biking. She recently participated in a mountain biking excursion through the Adirondack Mountains.

FAMILY HISTORY

Her mother, age 72, suffered a mild stroke 2 years ago with the temporary loss of function of her right leg. She has hypertension and has recovered all function of her leg. Her father, age 70, has mild diabetes. She has a 56-year-old brother with hypertension.

SEXUAL HISTORY

She has noted less frequent periods for the past year. She is sexually active with only her husband. She enjoys having sexual relations about once a week.

REVIEW OF SYSTEMS

Noncontributory

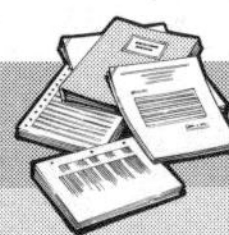

SP's Data Gathering (DG) Checklists

HISTORY CHECKLIST

1. I am a secretary.
2. I've been having severe pain in my left wrist and fingers.
3. The pain has gotten worse in my left wrist over the past 3 weeks.
4. There is numbness and burning of the fourth and fifth fingers of my left hand.
5. I recently noticed a sensory loss in the same fingers.
6. For the past week, I have noted an inability to use my left hand to button or unbutton my clothing.
7. I use a computer mouse with my right hand.
8. There is no tingling in the left arm or neck.
9. I am unaware of anything that makes it better or worse.
10. I have no difficulty with my speech.
11. I have no difficulty with my vision.
12. I have mild hypertension and high cholesterol.
13. I have no history of rheumatoid arthritis
14. I have no history of diabetes.
15. I have no history of thyroid disease.
16. I take atenolol 50 mg daily for hypertension and Lipitor 20 mg daily for high cholesterol.
17. I do not drink alcohol or use any other recreational drugs.
18. I enjoy yoga and mountain biking.
19. I recently participated in a mountain biking excursion through the Adirondack Mountains.
20. My mother suffered a mild stroke 2 years ago with the temporary loss of function of her right leg.
21. I have an allergy to shellfish and get a rash.

PHYSICAL CHECKLIST

1. Tested muscle strength in upper arms
2. Tested muscle strength in lower arms
3. Tested muscle strength in fingers
4. Tested sharp and dull sensation in fingers
5. Tapped over left wrist (Tinel's sign)
6. Tested DTRs of upper extremities

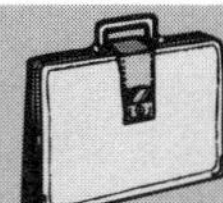

SP's Communication and Interpersonal Skills (CIS) Checklist

1. Knocked before entering
2. Opened interview by introducing self
3. Addressed patient using last name with introduction (e.g., Ms. Manoff)
4. Appearance (e.g., clean and neat)
5. Allowed patient to express reason for seeking medical attention
6. Made comfortable eye contact
7. Did *not* use leading/biased questions (e.g., "You don't have..." or "You're not...")
8. Asked questions individually
9. Did *not* use the "Why" question
10. Concentrated and focused on patient's needs
11. Maintained comfortable and appropriate distance
12. Gave patient time to think and answer without interrupting
13. Used proper draping during physical exam
14. Did physical examination in an orderly manner
15. Summarized patient's condition (or asked patient to summarize)
16. Discussed diagnostic tests and/or next step in treatment in lay terms
17. Asked whether patient had other questions/concerns
18. Provided patient education/suggestions where appropriate
19. Did *not* give false assurances
20. Showed empathy

123 SP's Spoken English Proficiency (SEP) Rating Scale

	Poor	Fair	Good	Very Good	Excellent
1. Ability of *patient* to understand *candidate*	1	2	3	4	5
2. Ability of *candidate* to understand *patient*	1	2	3	4	5
3. Candidate is articulate	1	2	3	4	5
4. Words are pronounced correctly	1	2	3	4	5
5. Range of vocabulary and sentence structure	1	2	3	4	5
6. Stress, rhythm, and intonation	1	2	3	4	5
7. Grammar	1	2	3	4	5
8. Repair strategies	1	2	3	4	5

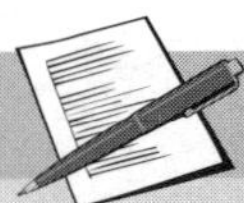

Example of a Satisfactory Patient Note (PN)

HISTORY—Include any significant pertinent positives and negatives

Ms. Judy Manoff is a 51-year-old secretary who presents to clinic for evaluation of progressive left wrist pain and numbness and burning of her fourth and fifth fingers of her left hand, which has developed over the past 3 weeks. She also describes a sensory loss in the same fingers. Over the past week, she has noted an inability to use her left hand to button or unbutton her clothing. She is extremely upset about her symptoms because she is right handed and uses the computer mouse with her right hand only. She is wondering why this is occurring in the hand she doesn't use as much. She is concerned that she might be having a stroke like her mother had several years ago. She denies tingling in the left arm or neck. She is unaware of anything that makes it better or worse. There is no history of difficulty in speech or in vision.

The patient has been in good health except for mild hypertension, treated with atenolol 50 mg daily, and high cholesterol, treated with Lipitor 20 mg daily. There is no history of rheumatoid arthritis, diabetes, or thyroid disease.

The patient is very athletic and enjoys mountain biking. She recently participated in a mountain biking excursion through the Adirondack Mountains.

PHYSICAL EXAMINATION—Include any significant pertinent positives and negatives

Physical examination reveals an anxious, well-developed, thin, 51-year-old woman appearing her stated age, and complaining of left wrist and hand pain. Vital signs are normal. Examination of the left hand reveals slight flexion of the fourth and fifth fingers. The patient is unable to abduct and adduct the fingers, and has very diminished strength in opposing the first and second fingers of the left hand. Muscle strength of the upper and lower left is within normal limits. There is decreased sensation to sharp and dull over the fourth and fifth fingers. A sharp tap over the left ulnar nerve at the wrist elicits paresthesia in the fourth and fifth left fingers. DTRs are normal.

DIFFERENTIAL DIAGNOSIS

In order of likelihood, write no more than five (5) differential diagnoses

1. Ganglion cyst with impingement on the ulnar nerve
2. Carpal tunnel syndrome
3. Ulnar neuropathy
4. Cervical radiculopathy
5. ____________________

DIAGNOSTIC WORKUP

Immediate plans, write no more than five (5) diagnostic studies

1. Nerve conduction velocity study
2. EMG
3. MRI of left wrist
4. CBC, Lyme antibody titer, ANA, ESR, RF
5. ____________________

CASE 5—Ms. Elizabeth Natt

Ms. Elizabeth Natt, a 39-year-old woman, presents to clinic complaining of numbness of her feet.

VITAL SIGNS

Temperature: 98.4° F	**Pulse:** 75 regular
Blood Pressure: 115/70	**Respiratory Rate:** 12 regular

EXAMINEE'S TASKS

In the next 15 minutes, you are to:

1) Take a focused history
2) Do a focused physical examination
3) Discuss your initial clinical impressions and workup plans with the patient
4) Write the Patient Note after leaving the room

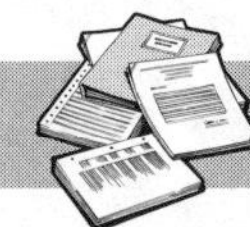

Examinee's Data Gathering (DG) Checklists

HISTORY CHECKLIST

1. ____
2. ____
3. ____
4. ____
5. ____
6. ____
7. ____
8. ____
9. ____
10. ____
11. ____
12. ____
13. ____
14. ____
15. ____
16. ____
17. ____
18. ____
19. ____
20. ____
21. ____

PHYSICAL EXAMINATION CHECKLIST

1. ____
2. ____
3. ____
4. ____
5. ____
6. ____

7. ______________________________
8. ______________________________

Total DG Score ______ *Passing Score for DG is 20 points (70%)*

Examinee's Communication and Interpersonal Skills (CIS) Checklist

1. ______________________________
2. ______________________________
3. ______________________________
4. ______________________________
5. ______________________________
6. ______________________________
7. ______________________________
8. ______________________________
9. ______________________________
10. ______________________________
11. ______________________________
12. ______________________________
13. ______________________________
14. ______________________________
15. ______________________________
16. ______________________________
17. ______________________________
18. ______________________________
19. ______________________________
20. ______________________________

Total CIS Score ______ *Passing Score for CIS is 14 points (70%)*

123 Examinee's Spoken English Proficiency (SEP) Rating Scale

	Poor	Fair	Good	Very Good	Excellent
1. Ability of *patient* to understand *candidate*	1	2	3	4	5
2. Ability of *candidate* to understand *patient*	1	2	3	4	5
3. Candidate is articulate	1	2	3	4	5
4. Words are pronounced correctly	1	2	3	4	5
5. Range of vocabulary and sentence structure	1	2	3	4	5
6. Stress, rhythm, and intonation	1	2	3	4	5
7. Grammar	1	2	3	4	5
8. Repair strategies	1	2	3	4	5

Total SEP Score ______ *Passing Score for SEP is 28 points (70%)*

Examinee's Patient Note (PN)

HISTORY—Include any significant pertinent positives and negatives

PHYSICAL EXAMINATION—Include any significant pertinent positives and negatives

DIFFERENTIAL DIAGNOSIS

In order of likelihood, write no more than five (5) differential diagnoses

1.
2.
3.
4.
5.

DIAGNOSTIC WORKUP

Immediate plans, write no more than five (5) diagnostic studies

1.
2.
3.
4.
5.

If you encounter an overtalkative patient, let them talk for 20–30 seconds and see what they have to say. If they are talking about inconsequential things, politely steer the conversation back to the issues at hand. If, on the other hand, as they are telling their story, you learn valuable information, let them talk on.

Background Information for Standardized Patient

PATIENT BEHAVIOR

Overtalkative; assumes that the symptoms are not important and transient.

AFFECT

Nice; hard for the doctor to get a word in edgewise; seems apologetic for concerning the doctor with this.

CHIEF COMPLAINT

"Numbness in my feet"

HISTORY OF PRESENT ILLNESS

Elizabeth Natt is a 39-year-old woman who presents to clinic for evaluation of numbness of both her feet. Over the past 2 months, the patient has noticed the onset of patchy loss of sensation in both her feet. She came to clinic today complaining of the feeling of "pins and needles," as well as areas of increased sensitivity. She also describes the sensation of "electric shocks" down her spine upon flexing her neck, beginning about 6 weeks ago.

PAST MEDICAL HISTORY

About 10 years ago, after the birth of her son Kevin, she developed the acute loss of vision in her right eye. There was a rapid loss of vision down to 20/200 followed by a complete restoration of vision within 6 weeks. During that period, she experienced pain on movement of the eye, as well as double vision. The double vision also resolved within the 6-week period. She was seen by an ophthalmologist at the time who diagnosed optic neuritis, and she was treated with steroids.

MEDICATIONS

None

ALLERGIES

None

SOCIAL HISTORY

She is married and lives with her husband and son. She is a housewife. She denies using any alcohol or other recreational drugs.

FAMILY HISTORY

Her mother is 60 years old and has diabetes, being treated by oral hypoglycemics. Her father is 62 years old and also has diabetes, being treated with insulin. Her older brother, age 42, has diabetes, being treated with insulin.

SEXUAL HISTORY

She is sexually active with only her husband, but has noted a decrease in desire to have sexual relations over the past few months. Her only pregnancy was complicated by an increase in weight gain, during which time her obstetrician told her she had developed gestational diabetes. At birth, Kevin weighed 10 pounds 2 ounces.

REVIEW OF SYSTEMS

There is no history of bowel or bladder problems.

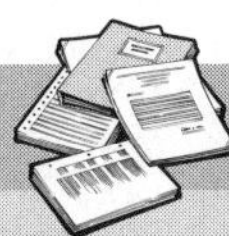

SP's Data Gathering (DG) Checklists

HISTORY CHECKLIST

1. I have numbness of both my feet
2. Over the past 2 months, I have noticed the onset of patchy loss of sensation in both my feet.
3. I came to clinic today because of the feeling of "pins and needles," as well as areas of increased sensitivity in my feet.
4. I noticed that about 6 weeks ago, I developed the sensation of "electric shocks" down my spine upon flexing my neck.
5. About 10 years ago, after the birth of my son Kevin, I developed the acute loss of vision in my right eye.
6. There was a rapid loss of vision down to 20/200.
7. It was followed by a complete restoration of vision within 6 weeks.
8. I experienced pain on movement of the right eye at that same time.
9. I also had double vision.
10. The double vision also resolved within the 6-week period.
11. I was seen by an ophthalmologist at this time who diagnosed optic neuritis.
12. I was treated with steroids for the optic neuritis.
13. There is no history of bowel or bladder problems.
14. I do not use any alcohol or other recreational drugs.
15. I do not take any medications.
16. I have no allergies.
17. My mother has diabetes.
18. My father has diabetes.
19. My older brother has diabetes.
20. When I was pregnant with my son, I developed gestational diabetes.
21. At birth, my son Kevin weighed 10 pounds 2 ounces.

PHYSICAL CHECKLIST

1. Mental status exam
2. Evaluated cranial nerves II, III, IV, and VI (vision and EOMs)—all required
3. Evaluated sharp and dull sensation in lower extremities
4. Tested DTRs in lower extremities
5. Evaluated cerebellar function with finger-to-nose or heel-to-shin test
6. Evaluated position sense in toes
7. Evaluated gait
8. Ophthalmoscopic examination

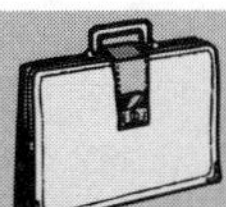

SP's Communication and Interpersonal Skills (CIS) Checklist

1. Knocked before entering
2. Opened interview by introducing self
3. Addressed patient using last name with introduction (e.g., Ms. Natt)
4. Appearance (e.g., clean and neat)
5. Allowed patient to express reason for seeking medical attention
6. Made comfortable eye contact
7. Did *not* use leading/biased questions (e.g., "You don't have…" or "You're not…")
8. Asked questions individually
9. Did *not* use the "Why" question
10. Concentrated and focused on patient's needs
11. Maintained comfortable and appropriate distance
12. Gave patient time to think and answer without interrupting
13. Used proper draping during physical exam
14. Did physical examination in an orderly manner
15. Summarized patient's condition (or asked patient to summarize)
16. Discussed diagnostic tests and/or next step in treatment in lay terms
17. Asked whether patient had other questions/concerns
18. Provided patient education/suggestions where appropriate
19. Did *not* give false assurances
20. Showed empathy

123 SP's Spoken English Proficiency (SEP) Rating Scale

	Poor	Fair	Good	Very Good	Excellent
1. Ability of *patient* to understand *candidate*	1	2	3	4	5
2. Ability of *candidate* to understand *patient*	1	2	3	4	5
3. Candidate is articulate	1	2	3	4	5
4. Words are pronounced correctly	1	2	3	4	5
5. Range of vocabulary and sentence structure	1	2	3	4	5
6. Stress, rhythm, and intonation	1	2	3	4	5
7. Grammar	1	2	3	4	5
8. Repair strategies	1	2	3	4	5

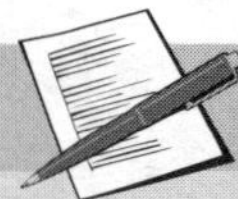

Example of a Satisfactory Patient Note (PN)

HISTORY—Include any significant pertinent positives and negatives

Ms. Elizabeth Natt is a 39-year-old, mother of one son, who presents to the clinic with the chief complaint of numbness of both her feet. Over the past 2 months, the patient has noticed the onset of patchy loss of sensation in both her feet. She came to clinic today complaining of the feeling of "pins and needles," as well as areas of increased sensitivity. She also describes the sensation of "electric shocks" down her spine upon flexing her neck, beginning about 6 weeks ago.

About 10 years ago, after the birth of her son Kevin, she developed the acute loss of vision in her right eye. There was a rapid loss of vision down to 20/200 followed by a complete restoration of vision within 6 weeks. During that period, she experienced pain on movement of the eye, as well as double vision. The double vision also resolved within the 6-week period. She was seen by an ophthalmologist at this time who diagnosed optic neuritis, and she was treated with steroids.

There is no history of bowel or bladder problems. The patient is not taking any medications and has no known allergies.

The patient lives with her husband and son. There is a strong family history of diabetes (mother, father, and older brother), as well as the patient having developed gestational diabetes with her son who was 10 pounds 2 ounces at birth.

PHYSICAL EXAMINATION—Include any significant pertinent positives and negatives

Physical examination reveals a well-developed, well-nourished, 39-year-old woman appearing her stated age, and complaining of numbness of her feet. Vital signs are normal. Ophthalmoscopic examination is within normal limits. The discs are pink with sharp margins, and the vasculature appears normal. The patient is oriented X3. Cranial nerves II, III, IV, and VI are intact. There is a loss of position sense and sharp/dull sensation in the toes of both feet. The DTRs are 4+ in the lower extremities with clonus present on the left. Cerebellar evaluation reveals a mild intention tremor on the left on finger-to-nose testing. Gait is normal.

DIFFERENTIAL DIAGNOSIS

In order of likelihood, write no more than five (5) differential diagnoses

1. Multiple sclerosis
2. R/O diabetes mellitus
3. R/O CNS vasculitis
4. R/O CNS tumor
5. R/O Conversion disorder

DIAGNOSTIC WORKUP

Immediate plans, write no more than five (5) diagnostic studies

1. Lumbar puncture and CSF analysis
2. CBC, ESR, glucose, hemoglobin A_{1C}
3. MRI of brain and spinal cord with contrast
4. ______
5. ______

CASE 6—Mr. Andrew Litt

Mr. Andrew Litt, a 27-year-old man, presents to clinic complaining of "the worst headache in his life."

VITAL SIGNS

Temperature: 99.8° F	**Pulse:** 95 regular
Blood Pressure: 160/90	**Respiratory Rate:** 14 regular

EXAMINEE'S TASKS

In the next 15 minutes, you are to:

1) Take a focused history
2) Do a focused physical examination
3) Discuss your initial clinical impressions and workup plans with the patient
4) Write the Patient Note after leaving the room

Examinee's Data Gathering (DG) Checklists

HISTORY CHECKLIST

1. ______
2. ______
3. ______
4. ______
5. ______
6. ______
7. ______
8. ______
9. ______
10. ______
11. ______
12. ______
13. ______
14. ______
15. ______
16. ______
17. ______
18. ______
19. ______
20. ______
21. ______
22. ______
23. ______

PHYSICAL EXAMINATION CHECKLIST

1. ______
2. ______
3. ______
4. ______
5. ______

6. ______________________________
7. ______________________________
8. ______________________________

Total DG Score ______ *Passing Score for DG is 22 points (70%)*

Examinee's Communication and Interpersonal Skills (CIS) Checklist

1. ______________________________
2. ______________________________
3. ______________________________
4. ______________________________
5. ______________________________
6. ______________________________
7. ______________________________
8. ______________________________
9. ______________________________
10. ______________________________
11. ______________________________
12. ______________________________
13. ______________________________
14. ______________________________
15. ______________________________
16. ______________________________
17. ______________________________
18. ______________________________
19. ______________________________
20. ______________________________

Total CIS Score ______ *Passing Score for CIS is 14 points (70%)*

123 Examinee's Spoken English Proficiency (SEP) Rating Scale

	Poor	Fair	Good	Very Good	Excellent
1. Ability of *patient* to understand *candidate*	1	2	3	4	5
2. Ability of *candidate* to understand *patient*	1	2	3	4	5
3. Candidate is articulate	1	2	3	4	5
4. Words are pronounced correctly	1	2	3	4	5
5. Range of vocabulary and sentence structure	1	2	3	4	5
6. Stress, rhythm, and intonation	1	2	3	4	5
7. Grammar	1	2	3	4	5
8. Repair strategies	1	2	3	4	5

Total SEP Score ______ *Passing Score for SEP is 28 points (70%)*

Examinee's Patient Note (PN)

HISTORY—Include any significant pertinent positives and negatives

PHYSICAL EXAMINATION—Include any significant pertinent positives and negatives

DIFFERENTIAL DIAGNOSIS

In order of likelihood, write no more than five (5) differential diagnoses

1.
2.
3.
4.
5.

DIAGNOSTIC WORKUP

Immediate plans, write no more than five (5) diagnostic studies

1.
2.
3.
4.
5.

Background Information for Standardized Patient

PATIENT BEHAVIOR

Does not readily move his head

AFFECT

Jittery, nervous

PROVOCATIVE QUESTION(S) AND PLAUSIBLE ANSWER(S)

"I know what migraines are, and this has got to be something else. Could I have a brain tumor?"

"Let's not jump to conclusions. I am going to ask you some questions and do a physical exam. Then we will see what is causing your severe pain."

CHIEF COMPLAINT

"This is the worst headache I've ever had."

HISTORY OF PRESENT ILLNESS

Andrew Litt is a 27-year-old man who presents to the emergency room for evaluation of "the worst headache" he has ever had. He states that the headache began about 30 hours ago and has gotten progressively worse. The pain is intense all over his head, especially behind his eyes. Over the past 5–6 hours, he noted that movement makes it worse. It is associated with severe nausea, and he has vomited several times. He has eye pain upon exposure to light. He denies a loss of consciousness, head trauma, preceding aura, or occurrence of seizures.

During the past week, his 3-year-old daughter and wife have been sick with a flulike illness associated with a runny nose and nasal congestion. Although he has not taken his temperature, he thinks he might have a fever.

He tried taking Fiorinal and acetaminophen, but there was minimal relief from the headache.

PAST MEDICAL HISTORY

He has a history of migraines for the past 10 years; the migraines occur about 3–4 times a year. They occur behind the left eye, without warning, last about 24 hours, and are relieved by Fiorinal tablets and rest. There is usually a preceding aura consisting of visual changes or loss of vision. He has noted that they are triggered by diet, emotional stress, or sleep deprivation.

He has high blood pressure, which is well controlled by medication.

MEDICATIONS
Atenolol 50 mg daily for hypertension; Fiorinal for headache as needed.

ALLERGIES
Bee stings (hives)

SOCIAL HISTORY
He has been married for 4 years and lives with his wife and daughter. He admits to drinking wine or beer daily with his wife, and he occasionally uses cocaine. He last used cocaine about 3 days ago.

FAMILY HISTORY
His parents are alive and well and have no chronic illnesses. He has two older brothers who are alive and well.

SEXUAL HISTORY
The patient is monogamous with his wife and enjoys sexual relations daily.

REVIEW OF SYSTEMS
Noncontributory

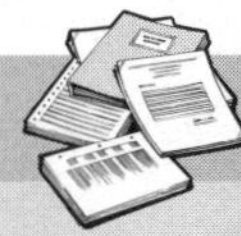

SP's Data Gathering (DG) Checklists

HISTORY CHECKLIST

1. My headache started about 30 hours ago.
2. It has gotten progressively worse.
3. I noticed that moving my head makes it worse.
4. I have severe nausea.
5. I vomited several times.
6. I have eye pain when I look at light.
7. I have not lost consciousness.
8. I have not had any head injury.
9. I have not had any seizures.
10. My daughter and my wife have been sick with a flulike illness in the past week.
11. They have a runny nose and nasal congestion.
12. I might have a fever.
13. I have taken Fiorinal and acetaminophen without much relief.
14. I have a history of migraines for the past 10 years.
15. The migraines occur behind the left eye, without warning, and last about 24 hours.
16. The migraines are relieved by Fiorinal tablets and rest.
17. The migraines usually have a preceding aura of visual changes or loss of vision.
18. The migraines are triggered by diet, emotional stress, or lack of sleep.
19. I have high blood pressure.
20. I take atenolol 50 mg daily for high blood pressure.
21. I occasionally use cocaine.
22. I last used cocaine about 3 days ago.
23. I am allergic to bee stings. I get hives.

PHYSICAL CHECKLIST

1. Took blood pressure
2. Evaluated EOMs
3. Evaluated pupillary reflexes
4. Performed ophthalmoscopic examination
5. Evaluated gross sensory function
6. Evaluated gross motor function
7. Tested for Kernig's and/or Brudzinski's signs
8. Performed auscultation of posterior lung fields

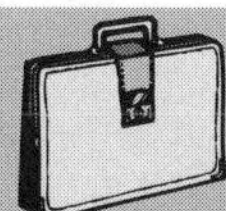

SP's Communication and Interpersonal Skills (CIS) Checklist

1. Knocked before entering
2. Opened interview by introducing self
3. Addressed patient using last name with introduction (e.g., Mr. Litt)
4. Appearance (e.g., clean and neat)
5. Allowed patient to express reason for seeking medical attention
6. Made comfortable eye contact
7. Did *not* use leading/biased questions (e.g., "You don't have..." or "You're not...")
8. Asked questions individually
9. Did *not* use the "Why" question
10. Concentrated and focused on patient's needs
11. Maintained comfortable and appropriate distance
12. Gave patient time to think and answer without interrupting
13. Used proper draping during physical exam
14. Did physical examination in an orderly manner
15. Summarized patient's condition (or asked patient to summarize)
16. Discussed diagnostic tests and/or next step in treatment in lay terms
17. Asked whether patient had other questions/concerns
18. Provided patient education/suggestions where appropriate
19. Did *not* give false assurances
20. Showed empathy

123 SP's Spoken English Proficiency (SEP) Rating Scale

	Poor	Fair	Good	Very Good	Excellent
1. Ability of *patient* to understand *candidate*	1	2	3	4	5
2. Ability of *candidate* to understand *patient*	1	2	3	4	5
3. Candidate is articulate	1	2	3	4	5
4. Words are pronounced correctly	1	2	3	4	5
5. Range of vocabulary and sentence structure	1	2	3	4	5
6. Stress, rhythm, and intonation	1	2	3	4	5
7. Grammar	1	2	3	4	5
8. Repair strategies	1	2	3	4	5

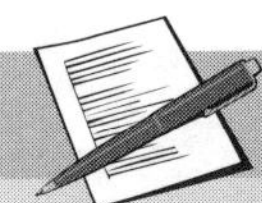

Example of a Satisfactory Patient Note (PN)

HISTORY—Include any significant pertinent positives and negatives

Mr. Andrew Litt is a 27-year-old man with a long history of migraine headaches who presents to the emergency room with "the worst headache in his life." The patient states that the headache began about 30 hours ago and has gotten progressively worse. Over the past 5–6 hours, he noted that movement makes it worse. It is associated with severe nausea, and he has vomited several times. He has eye pain upon exposure to light. He denies a loss of consciousness, head trauma, or occurrence of seizures. During the past week, his 3-year-old daughter and wife have been sick with a flulike illness associated with a runny nose and nasal congestion. Although he has not taken his temperature, he thinks he might have a fever.

He tried taking Fiorinal and acetaminophen, but there was minimal relief from the headache.

The patient has a 10-year history of migraine headaches, which occur about 3–4 times a year. They occur behind the left eye, without warning, last about 24 hours, and are relieved by Fiorinal tablets and rest. There is usually a preceding aura, usually composed of visual changes or scotomata. The patient has noted that the migraines are triggered by diet, emotional stress, or sleep deprivation.

The patient has a history of hypertension, well controlled by atenolol 50 mg daily. The patient has an "allergy" to bee stings manifested by hives. The patient admits to using cocaine occasionally; the last time was about 3 days ago.

PHYSICAL EXAMINATION—Include any significant pertinent positives and negatives

Physical examination reveals a lethargic but oriented X3, well-developed, well-nourished, 27-year-old man holding his head and complaining of a severe headache. Vital signs reveal a BP of 160/90. There is no evidence of head trauma. PERRL. EOMs are intact. Ophthalmoscopic examination is difficult because of the photophobia, but the disc margins appear sharp and the vasculature are WNL. Moderate nuchal rigidity is present at the extreme range of flexion and extension. Brudzinski's sign (leg hip flexion when the neck is flexed) is present. The chest is clear to percussion and auscultation. Gross sensory and motor functions are intact.

DIFFERENTIAL DIAGNOSIS

In order of likelihood, write no more than five (5) differential diagnoses

1. Meningitis
2. Migraine headache
3. Subarachnoid hemorrhage
4. Ruptured berry aneurysm
5. Cocaine-induced intracranial hemorrhage

DIAGNOSTIC WORKUP

Immediate plans, write no more than five (5) diagnostic studies

1. Lumbar puncture with CSF cultures
2. CBC, Lyme antibody titer, PT, PTT, blood cultures
3. CT scan of head
4. MRI/MRA if CT is negative
5. ______________________________

CASE 7—Mr. Charles Lang

Mr. Charles Lang, a 58-year-old man, presents to clinic complaining of progressive shortness of breath.

VITAL SIGNS

Temperature: 98.6° F	**Pulse:** 90 regular
Blood Pressure: 150/90	**Respiratory Rate:** 18 regular

EXAMINEE'S TASKS

In the next 15 minutes, you are to:

1. Take a focused history
2. Do a focused physical examination
3. Discuss your initial clinical impressions and workup plans with the patient
4. Write the Patient Note after leaving the room

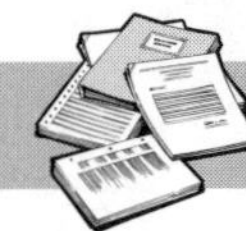

Examinee's Data Gathering (DG) Checklists

HISTORY CHECKLIST

1. ______
2. ______
3. ______
4. ______
5. ______
6. ______
7. ______
8. ______
9. ______
10. ______
11. ______
12. ______
13. ______
14. ______
15. ______
16. ______
17. ______
18. ______
19. ______
20. ______

PHYSICAL EXAMINATION CHECKLIST

1. ______
2. ______
3. ______
4. ______
5. ______
6. ______

7. ______________________________
8. ______________________________

Total DG Score _____ *Passing Score for DG is 20 points (70%)*

Examinee's Communication and Interpersonal Skills (CIS) Checklist

1. ______________________________
2. ______________________________
3. ______________________________
4. ______________________________
5. ______________________________
6. ______________________________
7. ______________________________
8. ______________________________
9. ______________________________
10. ______________________________
11. ______________________________
12. ______________________________
13. ______________________________
14. ______________________________
15. ______________________________
16. ______________________________
17. ______________________________
18. ______________________________
19. ______________________________
20. ______________________________

Total CIS Score _____ *Passing Score for CIS is 14 points (70%)*

123 Examinee's Spoken English Proficiency (SEP) Rating Scale

	Poor	Fair	Good	Very Good	Excellent
1. Ability of *patient* to understand *candidate*	1	2	3	4	5
2. Ability of *candidate* to understand *patient*	1	2	3	4	5
3. Candidate is articulate	1	2	3	4	5
4. Words are pronounced correctly	1	2	3	4	5
5. Range of vocabulary and sentence structure	1	2	3	4	5
6. Stress, rhythm, and intonation	1	2	3	4	5
7. Grammar	1	2	3	4	5
8. Repair strategies	1	2	3	4	5

Total SEP Score ______ *Passing Score for SEP is 28 points (70%)*

Examinee's Patient Note (PN)

HISTORY— Include any significant pertinent positives and negatives

PHYSICAL EXAMINATION—Include any significant pertinent positives and negatives

DIFFERENTIAL DIAGNOSIS

In order of likelihood, write no more than five (5) differential diagnoses

1.
2.
3.
4.
5.

DIAGNOSTIC WORKUP

Immediate plans, write no more than five (5) diagnostic studies

1.
2.
3.
4.
5.

Patients and doctors are partners in the patient's medical care. Although you have the medical knowledge essential to help the patient, the patient contributes because the patient knows him-/herself the best.

Background Information for Standardized Patient

PATIENT BEHAVIOR

Nothing out of the ordinary

AFFECT

Relaxed, congenial, but concerned

PROVOCATIVE QUESTION(S) AND PLAUSIBLE ANSWER(S)

"This couldn't be serious, could it?"

"It is too soon to tell. After the interview and a physical exam, I will know more."

CHIEF COMPLAINT

"It's been getting harder and harder to breathe."

HISTORY OF PRESENT ILLNESS

Charles Lang is a 58-year-old man who comes to clinic for evaluation of worsening shortness of breath for the past 2–3 years. He first noticed it at work, where he is physically pretty active, but now it bothers him even at rest. He does cough, but he does not bring up any sputum. He has never coughed up blood. Sometimes after coughing a lot, he might wheeze a little. He has never had chest pain except after a coughing fit. He also has had a 25-pound weight loss in the past 3–4 months. He was not trying to lose weight. He tries to eat normally, but his appetite is definitely less than about 6 months ago. He does not have any fever or chills, but he has had some frequent night sweats, waking up in sweat-soaked pajamas in the past few weeks. He is a 2-pack-per-day smoker for the past 30 years. He says that he knows he should stop, but he just can't do it!

PAST MEDICAL HISTORY

He has a 25-year history of high blood pressure, poorly controlled with medications.

MEDICATIONS

Atenolol 100 mg daily for high blood pressure
Aspirin

ALLERGIES

None

SOCIAL HISTORY

He has been a construction worker all his life. When he was 19 years old, he started working for a demolition company and worked with them for about 12 years before he started his own company. He now is thinking of selling his business because of his shortness of breath, which makes it difficult to work. He enjoys having 2–3 six-packs of beer per week with the guys.

FAMILY HISTORY

He has been married for the past 26 years and has four sons. His parents are both gone: mother died of a stroke (age 67) and father died of emphysema (age 60).

SEXUAL HISTORY

He has not been sexually active for the past 6 months because of his shortness of breath. He had two extramarital relationships several years ago.

REVIEW OF SYSTEMS

He has noted difficulty with urination for the past 2 years. The stream is not as forceful as it used to be, and he awakens nightly to urinate.

SP's Data Gathering (DG) Checklists

HISTORY CHECKLIST

1. It's been getting harder and harder to breath.
2. I have been getting more shortness of breath in the past 2–3 years.
3. I first noted the shortness of breath at work, but now I have it even at rest.
4. I cough a lot.
5. I do not bring up any sputum.
6. I have never coughed up blood.
7. Sometimes after coughing a lot, I wheeze a little.
8. I have never had chest pain except after a coughing fit.
9. I have had a 25-pound weight loss in the past 3–4 months.
10. I have not been trying to lose weight.
11. My appetite is definitely less than about 6 months ago.
12. I have not had fever or chills.
13. I have had some frequent night sweats waking me up in sweat-soaked pajamas in the past few weeks.
14. I am a 2-pack-per-day smoker for the past 30 years.
15. I've had high blood pressure for the past 25 years.
16. I take atenolol 100 mg daily for my high blood pressure.
17. I have no allergies.
18. I've been a construction worker all my life.
19. I worked there for about 12 years before I started my own company.
20. My father died of emphysema at age 60.

PHYSICAL CHECKLIST

1. Took blood pressure
2. Evaluated axillary lymphadenopathy by palpation
3. Evaluated anterior chest by percussion (4 places)
4. Evaluated anterior chest by auscultation (4 places)
5. Evaluated posterior chest by percussion (4 places)
6. Evaluated posterior chest by auscultation (4 places)
7. Evaluated cardiac PMI by palpation
8. Evaluated heart by auscultation (4 places)
7. Evaluated liver by palpation
8. Evaluated fingers and/or toes for clubbing

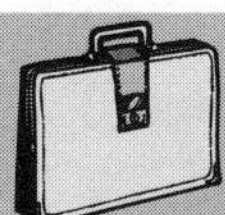

SP's Communication and Interpersonal Skills (CIS) Checklist

1. Knocked before entering
2. Opened interview by introducing self
3. Addressed patient using last name with introduction (e.g., Mr. Lang)
4. Appearance (e.g., clean and neat)
5. Allowed patient to express reason for seeking medical attention
6. Made comfortable eye contact
7. Did *not* use leading/biased questions (e.g., "You don't have..." or "You're not...")
8. Asked questions individually
9. Did *not* use the "Why" question
10. Concentrated and focused on patient's needs
11. Maintained comfortable and appropriate distance
12. Gave patient time to think and answer without interrupting
13. Used proper draping during physical exam
14. Did physical examination in an orderly manner
15. Summarized patient's condition (or asked patient to summarize)
16. Discussed diagnostic tests and/or next step in treatment in lay terms
17. Asked whether patient had other questions/concerns
18. Provided patient education/suggestions where appropriate
19. Did *not* give false assurances
20. Showed empathy

123 SP's Spoken English Proficiency (SEP) Rating Scale

	Poor	Fair	Good	Very Good	Excellent
1. Ability of *patient* to understand *candidate*	1	2	3	4	5
2. Ability of *candidate* to understand *patient*	1	2	3	4	5
3. Candidate is articulate	1	2	3	4	5
4. Words are pronounced correctly	1	2	3	4	5
5. Range of vocabulary and sentence structure	1	2	3	4	5
6. Stress, rhythm, and intonation	1	2	3	4	5
7. Grammar	1	2	3	4	5
8. Repair strategies	1	2	3	4	5

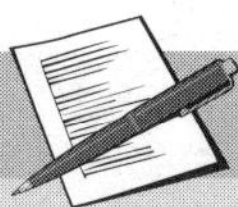

Example of a Satisfactory Patient Note (PN)

HISTORY—Include any significant pertinent positives and negatives

Mr. Charles Lang is a 58-year-old smoker (2 ppd × 30 years) and construction worker who comes to clinic for progressive shortness of breath over the past 2–3 years. He first noted it at work with exercise, but he now complains of it even at rest. The patient complains of a nonproductive cough and has never coughed up blood. On occasion, after a bout of coughing, the patient has noticed that he was wheezing. The patient denies chest pain except after a coughing spell. The patient relates that he has had a 25-pound weight loss in the past 3–4 months. His appetite is definitely less than about 6 months ago, but he still tries to eat as normally as possible. The patient does not have a history of any fever or chills, but in the past few weeks, he has had some frequent night sweats waking him up in sweat-soaked pajamas.

The patient has been in the building industry all his life. His first job at age 19 was with a demolition company with whom he had worked for 12 years before he started his own company. The patient has a 25-year history of high blood pressure, poorly controlled with atenolol 100 mg daily. He has no known allergies.

His father died of emphysema at age 60.

PHYSICAL EXAMINATION—Include any significant pertinent positives and negatives

Physical examination reveals a well-developed, thin, 58-year-old man appearing older than his stated age in moderate respiratory distress. BP is 155/90. There is labored breathing at a rate of 18/minute. No clubbing is present. No axillary lymphadenopathy is present. Evaluation of the posterior chest reveals a pleural rub at the level of the right lower scapula. A distinct wheeze is heard at that same location. Mild pulmonary crackles are heard throughout the lung fields. The PMI is subxiphoid. S_1S_2 are WNL. There are no murmurs, gallops, or pericardial rubs heard. The liver span is 14 cm in the midclavicular line.

DIFFERENTIAL DIAGNOSIS

In order of likelihood, write no more than five (5) differential diagnoses

1. Mesothelioma
2. Asbestosis
3. Lung cancer
4. COPD
5. Pleural fibrosis

DIAGNOSTIC WORKUP

Immediate plans, write no more than five (5) diagnostic studies

1. Chest x-ray
2. CBC, arterial blood gas, CO_2, ALT, AST, alkaline phosphatase, bilirubin
3. CT scan of chest
4. Pulmonary function tests
5. Bronchoscopy with biopsy pending above studies

CASE 8—Ms. Andrea Hill

Ms. Andrea Hill, a 34-year-old woman, presents to the Emergency Room complaining of chest pain.

VITAL SIGNS

Temperature: 98.4° F	**Pulse:** 75 regular
Blood Pressure: 115/65	**Respiratory Rate:** 12 regular

EXAMINEE'S TASKS

In the next 15 minutes, you are to:

1. Take a focused history
2. Do a focused physical examination
3. Discuss your initial clinical impressions and workup plans with the patient
4. Write the Patient Note after leaving the room

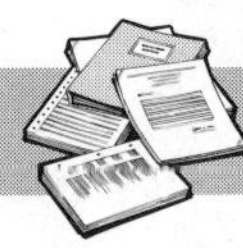

Examinee's Data Gathering (DG) Checklists

HISTORY CHECKLIST

1. ______
2. ______
3. ______
4. ______
5. ______
6. ______
7. ______
8. ______
9. ______
10. ______
11. ______
12. ______
13. ______
14. ______
15. ______
16. ______
17. ______
18. ______
19. ______
20. ______
21. ______
22. ______
23. ______

PHYSICAL EXAMINATION CHECKLIST

1. ______
2. ______
3. ______
4. ______

5. ______________________________
6. ______________________________

Total DG Score ______ *Passing Score for DG is 20 points (70%)*

Examinee's Communication and Interpersonal Skills (CIS) Checklist

1. ______________________________
2. ______________________________
3. ______________________________
4. ______________________________
5. ______________________________
6. ______________________________
7. ______________________________
8. ______________________________
9. ______________________________
10. ______________________________
11. ______________________________
12. ______________________________
13. ______________________________
14. ______________________________
15. ______________________________
16. ______________________________
17. ______________________________
18. ______________________________
19. ______________________________
20. ______________________________

Total CIS Score ______ *Passing Score for CIS is 14 points (70%)*

123 Examinee's Spoken English Proficiency (SEP) Rating Scale

	Poor	Fair	Good	Very Good	Excellent
1. Ability of *patient* to understand *candidate*	1	2	3	4	5
2. Ability of *candidate* to understand *patient*	1	2	3	4	5
3. Candidate is articulate	1	2	3	4	5
4. Words are pronounced correctly	1	2	3	4	5
5. Range of vocabulary and sentence structure	1	2	3	4	5
6. Stress, rhythm, and intonation	1	2	3	4	5
7. Grammar	1	2	3	4	5
8. Repair strategies	1	2	3	4	5

Total SEP Score ______ *Passing Score for SEP is 28 points (70%)*

Examinee's Patient Note (PN)

HISTORY—Include any significant pertinent positives and negatives

PHYSICAL EXAMINATION—Include any significant pertinent positives and negatives

DIFFERENTIAL DIAGNOSIS

In order of likelihood, write no more than five (5) differential diagnoses

1. ____
2. ____
3. ____
4. ____
5. ____

DIAGNOSTIC WORKUP

Immediate plans, write no more than five (5) diagnostic studies

1. ____
2. ____
3. ____
4. ____
5. ____

If you can unequivocally assure a patient that what they have is not the thing they are worrying about, do so. This is not false assurance.

Background Information for Standardized Patient

PATIENT BEHAVIOR

Tries to smile and act normal

AFFECT

Nervous, nice, deferential to the doctor

CHIEF COMPLAINT

"I think I'm having a heart attack."

HISTORY OF PRESENT ILLNESS

Andrea Hill is a 34-year-old woman who presents to clinic for evaluation of chest pain. She is very agitated and is worried that she is having a heart attack. She describes that the pain came on 2 hours ago, while she was reading a travel guide on Hawaii, where she and her husband are planning to visit next month. She has had this type of chest pain for the past 4 years. The pain is not related to exercise, anxiety, heavy meals, or sexual activity. The pain is very unpredictable, and she is unaware of what brings it on. Sometimes she has the pain every day, but sometimes she doesn't get it for a month. She describes the intensity of the pain today at about an 8 out of 10. The pain usually ranges in severity from 3 to 8. She describes the pain as very sharp in nature and is located directly in the center of her chest under her breastbone. The pain seems to get better by taking deep breaths and relaxing; it goes away in about an hour. The pain is not associated with shortness of breath, dizziness, palpitations, or sweating.

PAST MEDICAL HISTORY

She had Hashimoto's thyroiditis at age 18 and has been on thyroid replacement medication since age 23. Her cholesterol and sugar levels are normal.

MEDICATIONS

Synthroid 0.25 µg daily

ALLERGIES

None

SOCIAL HISTORY

The patient is a secretary at a law firm. She drinks 4–5 cups of regular coffee a day. She also enjoys chocolate, which she eats daily. She doesn't drink alcohol and has never used other recreational drugs. She has never smoked.

FAMILY HISTORY

She is happily married for the past 8 years. She has never been pregnant. She has been trying to get pregnant for the past 3 years, but has been unsuccessful. Her parents are both alive and in good health.

SEXUAL HISTORY

She is monogamous with her husband. Her periods are quite irregular. Her LMP was 2 weeks ago.

REVIEW OF SYSTEMS

Noncontributory

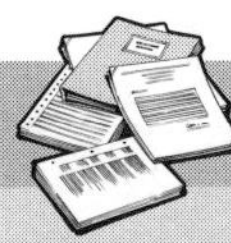

SP's Data Gathering (DG) Checklists

HISTORY CHECKLIST

1. I am worried that I'm having a heart attack.
2. The pain came on 2 hours ago, while I was reading a travel guide on Hawaii.
3. The pain is not related to exercise.
4. The pain is not related to anxiety.
5. The pain doesn't come on after heavy meals.
6. The pain is not related to sexual activity.
7. The pain is very unpredictable; I really don't know what brings it on.
8. Sometimes I get the pain every day, but sometimes I don't get it for a month.
9. Today, the intensity of the pain is about an 8 out of 10.
10. The pain ranges usually in severity from 3 to 8 out of 10.
11. The pain is very sharp in nature.
12. The pain is located directly in the center of my chest under my breastbone.
13. The pain seems to get better by taking deep breaths and relaxing.
14. The pain goes away in about an hour.
15. The pain is not associated with shortness of breath
16. The pain is not associated with dizziness.
17. The pain is not associated with palpitations.
18. The pain is not associated with sweating.
19. I had Hashimoto's thyroiditis at age 18.
20. I have been on thyroid replacement medications (Synthroid 25 µg daily) since age 23.
21. I drink about 4–5 cups of regular coffee a day.
22. I don't drink alcohol or use other recreational drugs.
23. I have no allergies.

PHYSICAL CHECKLIST

1. Took blood pressure
2. Palpated thyroid anteriorly and posteriorly
3. Palpated PMI
4. Evaluated heart by auscultation (4 areas)
5. Evaluated liver by palpation
6. Evaluated for peripheral edema

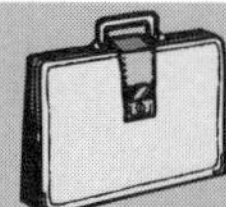

SP's Communication and Interpersonal Skills (CIS) Checklist

1. Knocked before entering
2. Opened interview by introducing self
3. Addressed patient using last name with introduction (e.g., Ms. Hill)
4. Appearance (e.g., clean and neat)
5. Allowed patient to express reason for seeking medical attention
6. Made comfortable eye contact
7. Did *not* use leading/biased questions (e.g., "You don't have…" or "You're not…")
8. Asked questions individually
9. Did *not* use the "Why" question
10. Concentrated and focused on patient's needs
11. Maintained comfortable and appropriate distance
12. Gave patient time to think and answer without interrupting
13. Used proper draping during physical exam
14. Did physical examination in an orderly manner
15. Summarized patient's condition (or asked patient to summarize)
16. Discussed diagnostic tests and/or next step in treatment in lay terms
17. Asked whether patient had other questions/concerns
18. Provided patient education/suggestions where appropriate
19. Did *not* give false assurances
20. Showed empathy

123 SP's Spoken English Proficiency (SEP) Rating Scale

	Poor	Fair	Good	Very Good	Excellent
1. Ability of *patient* to understand *candidate*	1	2	3	4	5
2. Ability of *candidate* to understand *patient*	1	2	3	4	5
3. Candidate is articulate	1	2	3	4	5
4. Words are pronounced correctly	1	2	3	4	5
5. Range of vocabulary and sentence structure	1	2	3	4	5
6. Stress, rhythm, and intonation	1	2	3	4	5
7. Grammar	1	2	3	4	5
8. Repair strategies	1	2	3	4	5

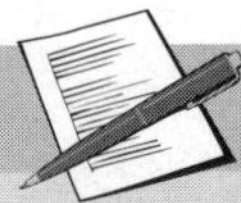

Example of a Satisfactory Patient Note (PN)

HISTORY—Include any significant pertinent positives and negatives

Ms. Andrea Hill is an anxious 34-year-old whose chief complaint is "I think I'm having a heart attack." She states that the pain began 2 hours ago, while she was reading a travel guide on Hawaii. The patient relates that she has had this type of chest pain for the past 4 years. The pain is atypical for coronary heart disease in that it is not related to exercise, anxiety, heavy meals, or sexual activity. The onset of the pain is very unpredictable. Sometimes the patient experiences chest pain every day, but sometimes she doesn't have it for a month. The patient states that today the intensity of the pain is about an 8 out of 10. At other times, the pain ranges in severity from 3 to 8. The retrosternal pain is described as very sharp in nature. The pain seems to get better by taking deep breaths and relaxing; it goes away in about an hour. The pain is not associated with shortness of breath, dizziness, palpitations, or sweating.

Past medical history is important in that the patient had Hashimoto's thyroiditis at age 18 and has been on Synthroid 0.25 μg daily since age 23. Her cholesterol and blood glucose have always been normal. The patient has no known allergies.

The patient is a secretary at a law firm and drinks 4–5 cups of regular coffee a day. She also enjoys chocolate, which she eats daily. The patient doesn't drink alcohol or use other recreational drugs. She has never smoked.

PHYSICAL EXAMINATION—Include any significant pertinent positives and negatives

Physical examination reveals an anxious, well-developed, thin, 34-year-old woman appearing her stated age, and complaining of retrosternal chest pain. BP is 120/60. Thyroid palpation reveals no abnormalities. The PMI is in the 5th ICS-MCL. S_1S_2 are WNL. There is a midsystolic click preceding a G II/VI late systolic murmur. The liver span is 10 cm in the midclavicular line; the edge is sharp. No peripheral edema is present.

DIFFERENTIAL DIAGNOSIS

In order of likelihood, write no more than five (5) differential diagnoses

1. Mitral valve prolapse
2. Panic disorder
3. Hypothyroidism
4. Hyperventilation syndrome
5. R/O CAD

DIAGNOSTIC WORKUP

Immediate plans, write no more than five (5) diagnostic studies

1. Echocardiogram
2. ECG
3. CBC, TSH, free T_4, cholesterol, CPK, lipid profile
4. Serial cardiac enzymes (troponin and CPK-MB)
5. Chest x-ray

CASE 9—Mr. Ted Fox

Mr. Ted Fox, a 63-year-old man, presents to clinic requesting a prescription refill for his blood pressure medications.

VITAL SIGNS

Temperature: 98.4° F	**Pulse:** 70 regular
Blood Pressure: 140/85	**Respiratory Rate:** 12 regular

EXAMINEE'S TASKS

In the next 15 minutes, you are to:

1) Take a focused history
2) Do a focused physical examination
3) Discuss your initial clinical impressions and workup plans with the patient
4) Write the Patient Note after leaving the room

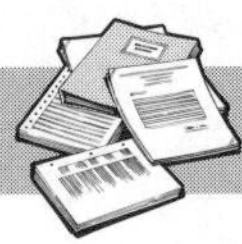

Examinee's Data Gathering (DG) Checklists

HISTORY CHECKLIST

1. ______
2. ______
3. ______
4. ______
5. ______
6. ______
7. ______
8. ______
9. ______
10. ______
11. ______
12. ______
13. ______
14. ______
15. ______
16. ______
17. ______
18. ______
19. ______
20. ______
21. ______
22. ______
23. ______
24. ______
25. ______

PHYSICAL EXAMINATION CHECKLIST

1. ______
2. ______
3. ______

4. ______________________________
5. ______________________________
6. ______________________________
7. ______________________________
8. ______________________________

Total DG Score ______ *Passing Score for DG is 23 points (70%)*

Examinee's Communication and Interpersonal Skills (CIS) Checklist

1. ______________________________
2. ______________________________
3. ______________________________
4. ______________________________
5. ______________________________
6. ______________________________
7. ______________________________
8. ______________________________
9. ______________________________
10. ______________________________
11. ______________________________
12. ______________________________
13. ______________________________
14. ______________________________
15. ______________________________
16. ______________________________
17. ______________________________
18. ______________________________
19. ______________________________
20. ______________________________

Total CIS Score ______ *Passing Score for CIS is 14 points (70%)*

123 Examinee's Spoken English Proficiency (SEP) Rating Scale

	Poor	Fair	Good	Very Good	Excellent
1. Ability of *patient* to understand *candidate*	1	2	3	4	5
2. Ability of *candidate* to understand *patient*	1	2	3	4	5
3. Candidate is articulate	1	2	3	4	5
4. Words are pronounced correctly	1	2	3	4	5
5. Range of vocabulary and sentence structure	1	2	3	4	5
6. Stress, rhythm, and intonation	1	2	3	4	5
7. Grammar	1	2	3	4	5
8. Repair strategies	1	2	3	4	5

Total SEP Score ______ *Passing Score for SEP is 28 points (70%)*

Examinee's Patient Note (PN)

HISTORY—Include any significant pertinent positives and negatives

PHYSICAL EXAMINATION— Include any significant pertinent positives and negatives

DIFFERENTIAL DIAGNOSIS

In order of likelihood, write no more than five (5) differential diagnoses

1.
2.
3.
4.
5.

DIAGNOSTIC WORKUP

Immediate plans, write no more than five (5) diagnostic studies

1.
2.
3.
4.
5.

Background Information for Standardized Patient

PATIENT BEHAVIOR

He just wants to get the prescription and leave.

AFFECT

Congenial

PROVOCATIVE QUESTION(S) AND PLAUSIBLE ANSWER(S)

"Why are you asking me all these questions about my sex life? I just want my prescription refilled."

"It's important to determine as it is possible that your decrease in sexual ability may be related to your medications."

ADDITIONAL NOTES

The patient doesn't want to talk about his erectile dysfunction and doesn't bring it up unless asked specifically about it. He then constantly tries to normalize it for his age.

If a patient seems impatient for no apparent reason, look at him/her carefully and listen carefully both to what is and isn't said, for clues to what might really be going on.

CHIEF COMPLAINT

"I need my blood pressure meds refilled. I would have done it over the phone, but they told me I needed to come in."

HISTORY OF PRESENT ILLNESS

Ted Fox is a 63-year-old man who presents to clinic for a prescription refill of his high blood pressure pills. His regular doctor, Dr. Kaiser, was called away for a family emergency. He is now being seen by one of Dr. Kaiser's associates whom he has not seen before. He's had high blood pressure for 16 years and has been on beta blockers for the whole time. He was first on propranolol, but was switched to atenolol about 8 years ago. His blood pressure seems to be under control. He also has had diabetes mellitus for the past 25 years and is now on insulin (35U NPH + 10U regular every morning). He had a "small" heart attack 3 years ago and was hospitalized for 7 days. He has had no significant chest pain since then, but he still fears having another episode; the first one was very scary.

PAST MEDICAL HISTORY

The patient had a basal cell cancer removed from his left forehead about 7 years ago. He has had no other surgery.

MEDICATIONS

Atenolol 100 mg daily
Aspirin
Insulin 35U NPH + 10U regular

ALLERGIES

None

SOCIAL HISTORY

He was an electrical engineer who retired 3 years ago. He used to smoke 2 packs per day but quit after his heart attack 3 years ago. He likes to drink wine with his meals, and enjoys red wine about 2–3 times a week.

FAMILY HISTORY

He has been married for the past 35 years. He has three children: a daughter, age 32, and two sons, ages 30 and 28. He has three grandchildren by his older son. His parents are deceased. His mother died at age 69 from diabetes, and his father died at age 76 from pneumonia and complications from a stroke. Recently, he learned that his daughter is using drugs, and he is very worried about it.

SEXUAL HISTORY

For the past 2–3 years, he has had gradual loss of ability to have sex with his wife. It seems to be getting worse. He loves his wife and has no other partners. He can get erections when sexually excited, but they are not as hard as several years ago, and he has difficulty maintaining them for penetration. He is still interested in having sexual relations, but he is not confident about his sexual activity. He still has morning erections which occur about 1–2 times a month. He masturbates in the shower occasionally; he can get an erection, and can ejaculate some of the time. He doesn't read pornographic magazines (nothing else sexually excites him). He has no hot/cold intolerance, tremor, visual disturbances, pain with sex, penile discharge, or weight changes.

REVIEW OF SYSTEMS

He has a small cataract in his left eye, but the doctor told him just to wait as his vision was still pretty good.

SP's Data Gathering (DG) Checklists

HISTORY CHECKLIST

1. I need to get my blood pressure meds refilled.
2. I've had high blood pressure for 16 years.
3. I've been on beta blockers for the whole time.
4. I was first treated with propranolol for about 8 years.
5. About 8 years ago, my doctor switched me to atenolol.
6. I have had diabetes mellitus for the past 25 years.
7. I am on insulin 35U NPH + 10U regular every morning.
8. I had a "small" heart attack 3 years ago.
9. I've had no significant chest pain since then.
10. I'm afraid that I might have another heart attack.
11. For the past 2–3 years, I've had difficulty having sex.
12. I love my wife and have had no other sexual partners.
13. I can get hard-ons (*slang for erections*) with sex, but they are not as hard as several years ago.
14. I have difficulty maintaining my hard-on for penetration.
15. I am still interested in having sexual relations.
16. I am not at all confident about my performance.
17. I still get morning hard-ons about 1–2 times a month.
18. I masturbate occasionally in the shower.
19. I do not have any hot/cold intolerance.
20. I do not have a tremor.
21. I am unaware of any visual disturbances.
22. I do not have pain with sex.
23. I recently learned that my daughter is using drugs.
24. I am very worried about it.
25. I have no allergies.

PHYSICAL CHECKLIST

1. Took blood pressure
2. Palpated carotids *after* auscultation
3. Tested visual fields by confrontation
4. Ophthalmoscopic examination
5. Palpated thyroid anteriorly and posteriorly

6. Examined heart by auscultation
7. Tested sensation in lower extremity
8. Tested vibration sense in lower extremity

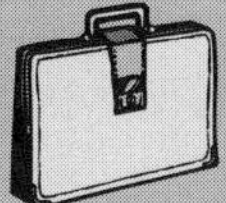

SP's Communication and Interpersonal Skills (CIS) Checklist

1. Knocked before entering
2. Opened interview by introducing self
3. Addressed patient using last name with introduction (e.g., Mr. Fox)
4. Appearance (e.g., clean and neat)
5. Allowed patient to express reason for seeking medical attention
6. Made comfortable eye contact
7. Did *not* use leading/biased questions (e.g., "You don't have..." or "You're not...")
8. Asked questions individually
9. Did *not* use the "Why" question
10. Concentrated and focused on patient's needs
11. Maintained comfortable and appropriate distance
12. Gave patient time to think and answer without interrupting
13. Used proper draping during physical exam
14. Did physical examination in an orderly manner
15. Summarized patient's condition (or asked patient to summarize)
16. Discussed diagnostic tests and/or next step in treatment in lay terms
17. Asked whether patient had other questions/concerns
18. Provided patient education/suggestions where appropriate
19. Did *not* give false assurances
20. Showed empathy

123 SP's Spoken English Proficiency (SEP) Rating Scale

	Poor	Fair	Good	Very Good	Excellent
1. Ability of *patient* to understand *candidate*	1	2	3	4	5
2. Ability of *candidate* to understand *patient*	1	2	3	4	5
3. Candidate is articulate	1	2	3	4	5
4. Words are pronounced correctly	1	2	3	4	5
5. Range of vocabulary and sentence structure	1	2	3	4	5
6. Stress, rhythm, and intonation	1	2	3	4	5
7. Grammar	1	2	3	4	5
8. Repair strategies	1	2	3	4	5

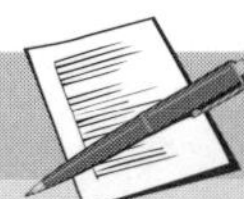

Example of a Satisfactory Patient Note (PN)

HISTORY—Include any significant pertinent positives and negatives

Mr. Ted Fox is a 63-year-old man who presents to clinic for a refill of atenolol 100 mg po daily for hypertension.

- H/O hypertension × 16 years (always on beta blockers alone)
- H/O diabetes mellitus × 25 years
- H/O MI 3 years ago—no chest pain since but worried that he'll have another MI

Upon questioning about adverse effects of the beta blocker, Mr. Fox reluctantly revealed that for the past 2–3 years, he's had ED which seems to be getting worse. He is able to have erections, but they are not as strong as several years ago, and he has difficulty maintaining it for penetration. His libido is still good, but he is not confident about his performance. He does relate that he still has morning erections about 1–2 times a month. He is able to masturbate occasionally in the shower. He states that nothing else sexually excites him. There are no symptoms of thyroid dysfunction (i.e., hot/cold intolerance or tremor). He is unaware of any visual disturbances. He has no pain with sex.

Recently he learned that his daughter is using drugs, and he is very concerned about it.

He has no allergies.

Meds: Atenolol 100 mg po daily

Insulin 35U NPH + 10U Regular

PHYSICAL EXAMINATION—Include any significant pertinent positives and negatives

Physical examination reveals a well-developed, slightly obese, 63-year-old man appearing slightly older than his stated age. BP is 145/85. Confrontational field testing reveals no abnormalities. Ophthalmoscopic exam of the right eye shows a normal-appearing disc. There are several microaneurysms near the macula. The left fundus is poorly visualized because of the small cataract, but it appears grossly normal. The carotids are full; no bruits are present. Examination of the thyroid by palpation is unremarkable. Examination of the heart reveals the PMI to be in the 5th ICS-MCL. S_1S_2 are WNL. There are no murmurs, gallops, or rubs present. There is decreased sensation to light touch on the left foot, which is a greater decrease than on the right. Vibration sense is intact.

DIFFERENTIAL DIAGNOSIS	**DIAGNOSTIC WORKUP**
In order of likelihood, write no more than five (5) differential diagnoses	Immediate plans, write no more than five (5) diagnostic studies
1. H/O hypertension, diabetes mellitus, CAD	1. Male GU exam
2. Drug-related erectile dysfunction (ED)	2. Rectal exam
3. R/O diabetes-related ED	3. CBC, fasting glucose, hemoglobin A_{1C}, serum testosterone, lipid panel, TSH, free T_4, prolactin
4. R/O hypothyroidism-related ED	4. Nocturnal penile tumescence testing
5. R/O psychogenic ED	5. Penile ultrasonography

CASE 10—Mr. David Evans

Mr. David Evans, a 52-year-old man, presents to clinic complaining of blood in his urine.

VITAL SIGNS

Temperature: 98.6° F	**Pulse:** 75 regular
Blood Pressure: 120/70	**Respiratory Rate:** 12 regular

EXAMINEE'S TASKS

In the next 15 minutes, you are to:

1. Take a focused history
2. Do a focused physical examination
3. Discuss your initial clinical impressions and workup plans with the patient
4. Write the Patient Note after leaving the room

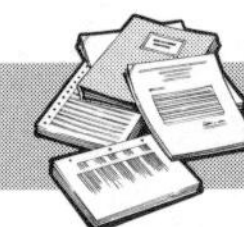

Examinee's Data Gathering (DG) Checklists

HISTORY CHECKLIST

1. ______
2. ______
3. ______
4. ______
5. ______
6. ______
7. ______
8. ______
9. ______
10. ______
11. ______
12. ______
13. ______
14. ______
15. ______
16. ______
17. ______
18. ______
19. ______
20. ______
21. ______
22. ______
23. ______

PHYSICAL EXAMINATION CHECKLIST

1. ______
2. ______
3. ______
4. ______

5. ______________________________
6. ______________________________

Total DG Score _____ *Passing Score for DG is 20 points (70%)*

Examinee's Communication and Interpersonal Skills (CIS) Checklist

1. ______________________________
2. ______________________________
3. ______________________________
4. ______________________________
5. ______________________________
6. ______________________________
7. ______________________________
8. ______________________________
9. ______________________________
10. ______________________________
11. ______________________________
12. ______________________________
13. ______________________________
14. ______________________________
15. ______________________________
16. ______________________________
17. ______________________________
18. ______________________________
19. ______________________________
20. ______________________________

Total CIS Score _____ *Passing Score for CIS is 14 points (70%)*

Examinee's Spoken English Proficiency (SEP) Rating Scale

	Poor	Fair	Good	Very Good	Excellent
1. Ability of *patient* to understand *candidate*	1	2	3	4	5
2. Ability of *candidate* to understand *patient*	1	2	3	4	5
3. Candidate is articulate	1	2	3	4	5
4. Words are pronounced correctly	1	2	3	4	5
5. Range of vocabulary and sentence structure	1	2	3	4	5
6. Stress, rhythm, and intonation	1	2	3	4	5
7. Grammar	1	2	3	4	5
8. Repair strategies	1	2	3	4	5

Total SEP Score ______ *Passing Score for SEP is 28 points (70%)*

Examinee's Patient Note (PN)

HISTORY—Include any significant pertinent positives and negatives

PHYSICAL EXAMINATION—Include any significant pertinent positives and negatives

DIFFERENTIAL DIAGNOSIS

In order of likelihood, write no more than five (5) differential diagnoses

1.
2.
3.
4.
5.

DIAGNOSTIC WORKUP

Immediate plans, write no more than five (5) diagnostic studies

1.
2.
3.
4.
5.

It is as important to appropriately assure the patient that he did the right thing by coming in so soon after he noticed this and to attempt to offer as much comfort and support to him as possible, as it is to diagnose what is wrong with him.

Background Information for Standardized Patient

PATIENT BEHAVIOR

In a hurry; keeps his answers short; nervous foot tapping; keeps checking his cell phone. Wants to call wife when he hears what he has.

AFFECT

Controlled panic

PROVOCATIVE QUESTION(S) AND PLAUSIBLE ANSWER(S)

"Do I have cancer?"

"It's too early to say. Let's get some tests done first, and then we will be in a better position to know."

CHIEF COMPLAINT

"I've got blood in my urine!"

HISTORY OF PRESENT ILLNESS

David Evans is a 52-year-old man who complains of 3 episodes of red urine over the past 24 hours. He got really scared this morning when he saw a blood clot in his urine and came for evaluation. When he first saw his red urine yesterday he thought that it was red because of the beet salad his wife had made for dinner the night before, but when it didn't clear up, he became very scared. He has never had this before. There is no burning on urination, urinary frequency, fever, night sweats, flank pain, or weight loss. He has never had kidney stones or familial kidney disease. He does not have nausea, vomiting, or diarrhea.

He has had an increasing need to awaken in the middle of the night to urinate. This started about a year ago. He also noticed that his stream is less forceful.

Two weeks ago, he ran in the city marathon and did very well. He wonders if that could be the cause of his red urine.

PAST MEDICAL HISTORY

He had an appendectomy at age 24.

MEDICATIONS

None

ALLERGIES

None

SOCIAL HISTORY
He is an accountant. He enjoys drinking single malt scotch with friends on the weekend. He was drunk only once in his life—in college. He smokes $1\frac{1}{2}$ ppd × 25 years. He has tried to quit, but just can't.

FAMILY HISTORY
He has been married to his second wife for the past 10 years. His first wife died in a car accident. He has two daughters from his first marriage. They are 18 and 20 years old. His mother, age 77, has diabetes. His father had a heart attack at age 60, but is now 79 and doing well.

SEXUAL HISTORY
He is sexually active with his wife only.

REVIEW OF SYSTEMS
Noncontributory

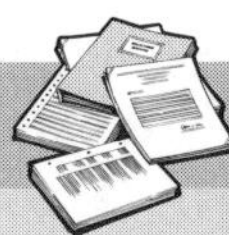

SP's Data Gathering (DG) Checklists

HISTORY CHECKLIST

1. "I've got blood in my urine!"
2. It started 24 hours ago.
3. I've had 3 episodes of red urine.
4. I saw a blood clot in my urine this morning.
5. When I first saw the red urine, I thought it was from my wife's beet salad the night before.
6. I have never had this before.
7. There is no burning on urination.
8. I don't urinate more frequently.
9. I do not have a fever.
10. I do not have night sweats.
11. I do not have flank pain.
12. I have not lost any weight.
13. I have never had kidney stones.
14. No one in my family has had kidney problems.
15. I do not have nausea or vomiting.
16. I do not have diarrhea.
17. I've been having to get up in the middle of the night to pee.
18. This started about a year ago.
19. I have noticed that my peeing is less forceful.
20. Two weeks ago, I ran in the city marathon.
21. I am not on any medications.
22. I have no allergies.
23. I smoke cigarettes, 1½ ppd × 25 years.

PHYSICAL CHECKLIST

1. Examined the anterior and posterior lung fields by auscultation
2. Examined the heart by auscultation
3. Performed light palpation of the abdomen in all 4 quadrants *after* auscultation
4. Performed deep palpation of the abdomen in all 4 quadrants
5. Percussed abdomen in all 4 quadrants
6. Checked for CVA tenderness

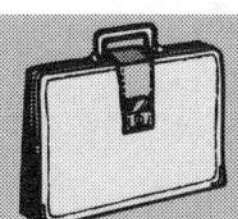

SP's Communication and Interpersonal Skills (CIS) Checklist

1. Knocked before entering
2. Opened interview by introducing self
3. Addressed patient using last name with introduction (e.g., Mr. Evans)
4. Appearance (e.g., clean and neat)
5. Allowed patient to express reason for seeking medical attention
6. Made comfortable eye contact
7. Did *not* use leading/biased questions (e.g., "You don't have..." or "You're not...")
8. Asked questions individually
9. Did *not* use the "Why" question
10. Concentrated and focused on patient's needs
11. Maintained comfortable and appropriate distance
12. Gave patient time to think and answer without interrupting
13. Used proper draping during physical exam
14. Did physical examination in an orderly manner
15. Summarized patient's condition (or asked patient to summarize)
16. Discussed diagnostic tests and/or next step in treatment in lay terms
17. Asked whether patient had other questions/concerns
18. Provided patient education/suggestions where appropriate
19. Did *not* give false assurances
20. Showed empathy

123 SP's Spoken English Proficiency (SEP) Rating Scale

	Poor	Fair	Good	Very Good	Excellent
1. Ability of *patient* to understand *candidate*	1	2	3	4	5
2. Ability of *candidate* to understand *patient*	1	2	3	4	5
3. Candidate is articulate	1	2	3	4	5
4. Words are pronounced correctly	1	2	3	4	5
5. Range of vocabulary and sentence structure	1	2	3	4	5
6. Stress, rhythm, and intonation	1	2	3	4	5
7. Grammar	1	2	3	4	5
8. Repair strategies	1	2	3	4	5

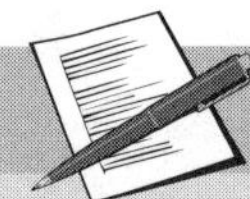

Example of a Satisfactory Patient Note (PN)

HISTORY—Include any significant pertinent positives and negatives

Mr. David Evans is a 52-year-old accountant who presents with the chief complaint of "I've got blood in my urine!"

HISTORY OF PRESENT ILLNESS

- Red urine started 24 hours ago
- Has had 3 episodes of red urine and a blood clot this morning
- No previous history of red urine
- No history of burning on urination, frequency, fever, night sweats, flank pain, or weight loss
- No history of kidney stones.
- No history of nausea, vomiting, or diarrhea
- One-year history of nocturia and weak stream
- Ran in city marathon 1 week ago

PAST MEDICAL HISTORY

- Appendectomy, age 24
- No medications
- No allergies

SOCIAL HISTORY

- Smokes cigarettes, $1\frac{1}{2}$ ppd × 25 years
- Drinks single malt scotch on weekends

FAMILY HISTORY

- Mother, age 77, diabetes
- Father, age 79, MI age 60
- Married 2nd time after 1st wife's accidental death
- Two daughters, ages 18 and 20
- No history of kidney problems

PHYSICAL EXAMINATION—Include any significant pertinent positives and negatives

GENERAL

- Physical examination reveals a well-developed, well-nourished, young-appearing, 52-year-old man

VITAL SIGNS

- BP 120/70
- Otherwise WNL

LUNGS

- Clear to P&A

HEART

- PMI 5th ICS-MCL
- S_1S_2 WNL
- (−) murmurs, gallops, or rubs

ABDOMEN

- scaphoid
- (+) bowel sounds
- (−) tenderness
- (−) masses
- (−) CVAT

DIFFERENTIAL DIAGNOSIS

In order of likelihood, write no more than five (5) differential diagnoses

1. Transitional cell bladder tumor
2. BPH
3. Cancer of the prostate
4. Renal cell carcinoma
5. Exertional hematuria

DIAGNOSTIC WORKUP

Immediate plans, write no more than five (5) diagnostic studies

1. Male GU & rectal exams
2. CBC, BUN, creatinine, PSA
3. U/A and urine for C/S
4. Ultrasound of prostate (transrectal)
5. CT of abdomen & pelvis

CASE 11—Mr. Sylvester Flint

Mr. Sylvester Flint, a 55-year-old man, presents to the emergency room complaining of dizziness.

VITAL SIGNS

Temperature: 98.8° F	**Pulse:** 90 regular
Blood Pressure: 130/70	**Respiratory Rate:** 14 regular

EXAMINEE'S TASKS

In the next 15 minutes, you are to:

1. Take a focused history
2. Do a focused physical examination
3. Discuss your initial clinical impressions and workup plans with the patient
4. Write the Patient Note after leaving the room

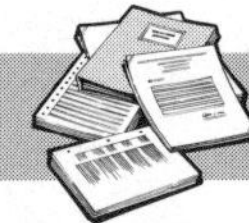

Examinee's Data Gathering (DG) Checklists

HISTORY CHECKLIST

1. ______
2. ______
3. ______
4. ______
5. ______
6. ______
7. ______
8. ______
9. ______
10. ______
11. ______
12. ______
13. ______
14. ______
15. ______
16. ______
17. ______
18. ______
19. ______

PHYSICAL EXAMINATION CHECKLIST

1. ______
2. ______
3. ______
4. ______
5. ______
6. ______
7. ______

Total DG Score ______ *Passing Score for DG is 18 points (70%)*

Examinee's Communication and Interpersonal Skills (CIS) Checklist

1. ______
2. ______
3. ______
4. ______
5. ______
6. ______
7. ______
8. ______
9. ______
10. ______
11. ______
12. ______
13. ______
14. ______
15. ______
16. ______
17. ______
18. ______
19. ______
20. ______

Total CIS Score ______ *Passing Score for CIS is 14 points (70%)*

123 Examinee's Spoken English Proficiency (SEP) Rating Scale

	Poor	Fair	Good	Very Good	Excellent
1. Ability of *patient* to understand *candidate*	1	2	3	4	5
2. Ability of *candidate* to understand *patient*	1	2	3	4	5
3. Candidate is articulate	1	2	3	4	5
4. Words are pronounced correctly	1	2	3	4	5
5. Range of vocabulary and sentence structure	1	2	3	4	5
6. Stress, rhythm, and intonation	1	2	3	4	5
7. Grammar	1	2	3	4	5
8. Repair strategies	1	2	3	4	5

Total SEP Score _____ *Passing Score for SEP is 28 points (70%)*

Examinee's Patient Note (PN)

HISTORY—Include any significant pertinent positives and negatives

PHYSICAL EXAMINATION—Include any significant pertinent positives and negatives

DIFFERENTIAL DIAGNOSIS

In order of likelihood, write no more than five (5) differential diagnoses

1.
2.
3.
4.
5.

DIAGNOSTIC WORKUP

Immediate plans, write no more than five (5) diagnostic studies

1.
2.
3.
4.
5.

Background Information for Standardized Patient

PATIENT BEHAVIOR
Eyes closed; holds his head very still with his hands; does not smile

AFFECT
Nervous; very anxious; extremely upset

PROVOCATIVE QUESTION(S) AND PLAUSIBLE ANSWER(S)
"Can you give me something immediately? I am so dizzy!"

"Let me first ask you some questions and do a few tests to determine what's going on. I promise you that I will give you something as soon as I have a better idea of your medical problem."

ADDITIONAL NOTES
Lying flat on stretcher; refuses to walk because he is so dizzy but will walk assisted if candidate explains the importance of the test.

CHIEF COMPLAINT
"Dizziness"

HISTORY OF PRESENT ILLNESS
Sylvester Flint is a 55-year-old man who comes to the emergency room for evaluation of severe dizziness. He states that the entire room is spinning. The sensation started yesterday morning after breakfast and has become progressively worse. Now it is almost constant, but initially it came in waves. It is worse when he tries to sit or stand up. Nothing seems to make it better except lying perfectly still. He has also had severe nausea and vomiting. He has vomited about 10 times. The vomit is yellow and does not have any blood in it. He noticed yesterday evening that he had some ringing in his ears and a maybe a little difficulty in hearing in his left ear, but he is not sure. He has no pressure or fullness sensation in his ears. He has no discharge from his ears. He has had no head injury. He thinks he may have had a fever but didn't take his temperature.

He had an upper respiratory infection with sneezing and a runny nose last week.

PAST MEDICAL HISTORY
He had a ruptured appendix when he was 36 and was really sick with peritonitis. He was on intravenous antibiotics for about 2 weeks. He thinks the drug was gentamicin.

MEDICATIONS
None

ALLERGIES
None

SOCIAL HISTORY
He is a mechanical engineer and works for a large company. He is married with one son, age 16. He drinks a "few beers a week" with the guys after work. He denies any other recreational drug use. In college, he tried acid and pot.

FAMILY HISTORY
His mother is 80 years old and has severe osteoarthritis and diabetes. His father died of lung cancer at age 70. He has an older brother with high blood pressure.

SEXUAL HISTORY
He had a history of syphilis when he was in college and was treated with penicillin. He married late in life after having many girlfriends. He is now monogamous with his wife.

REVIEW OF SYSTEMS
Noncontributory

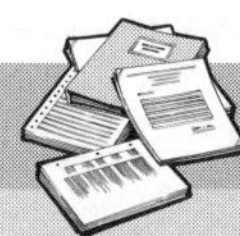

SP's Data Gathering (DG) Checklists

HISTORY CHECKLIST

1. The entire room is spinning.
2. The sensation started yesterday morning after breakfast and has become progressively worse.
3. Now it is almost constant, but initially it came in waves.
4. It is worse when I try to sit or stand up.
5. Nothing seems to make it better except lying perfectly still.
6. I have severe nausea and vomiting and vomited about 10 times.
7. The vomit is yellow in color.
8. There is no blood in it.
9. I had some ringing in my ears yesterday.
10. I may have a little difficulty in hearing in my left ear.
11. I do not have any pressure or fullness sensation in my ears.
12. I have no discharge from my ears.
13. I have never had any head injury.
14. I think I may have a fever.
15. I had an upper respiratory infection with sneezing and a runny nose last week.
16. I had a ruptured appendix when I was about 36 and was hospitalized and given intravenous antibiotics for about 2 weeks.
17. I am not on any medications.
18. I have no allergies.
19. I do not use recreational drugs.

PHYSICAL CHECKLIST

1. Took blood pressure
2. Evaluated EOMs
3. Performed an ophthalmoscopic examination
4. Evaluated external auditory canal and tympanic membranes
5. Assessed hearing with Weber and/or Rinne test
6. Assessed DTRs in lower extremities
7. Assessed gait

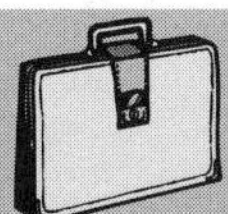

SP's Communication and Interpersonal Skills (CIS) Checklist

1. Knocked before entering
2. Opened interview by introducing self
3. Addressed patient using last name with introduction (e.g., Mr. Flint)
4. Appearance (e.g., clean and neat)
5. Allowed patient to express reason for seeking medical attention
6. Made comfortable eye contact
7. Did *not* use leading/biased questions (e.g., "You don't have…" or "You're not…")
8. Asked questions individually
9. Did *not* use the "Why" question
10. Concentrated and focused on patient's needs
11. Maintained comfortable and appropriate distance
12. Gave patient time to think and answer without interrupting
13. Used proper draping during physical exam
14. Did physical examination in an orderly manner
15. Summarized patient's condition (or asked patient to summarize)
16. Discussed diagnostic tests and/or next step in treatment in lay terms
17. Asked whether patient had other questions/concerns
18. Provided patient education/suggestions where appropriate
19. Did *not* give false assurances
20. Showed empathy

123 SP's Spoken English Proficiency (SEP) Rating Scale

	Poor	Fair	Good	Very Good	Excellent
1. Ability of *patient* to understand *candidate*	1	2	3	4	5
2. Ability of *candidate* to understand *patient*	1	2	3	4	5
3. Candidate is articulate	1	2	3	4	5
4. Words are pronounced correctly	1	2	3	4	5
5. Range of vocabulary and sentence structure	1	2	3	4	5
6. Stress, rhythm, and intonation	1	2	3	4	5
7. Grammar	1	2	3	4	5
8. Repair strategies	1	2	3	4	5

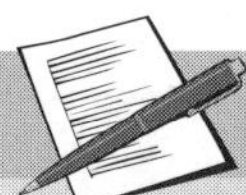

Example of a Satisfactory Patient Note (PN)

HISTORY—Include any significant pertinent positives and negatives

Mr. Sylvester Flint is a 55-year-old man who presents with "severe dizziness" to the ER.

HISTORY OF PRESENT ILLNESS

- Dizziness started yesterday after breakfast and has become progressively worse
- Initially in waves but now constant
- Worse when sitting or standing up and nothing seems to make it better except lying perfectly still
- (+) nausea for past 24 hours
- (+) vomited 10× in past 24 hours; yellow in color, no blood
- (+) warm (thinks he may have a fever)
- (+) ringing in ears yesterday with a little difficulty in hearing in left ear
- (+) H/O URI with sneezing and a runny nose last week
- (–) pressure or fullness sensation in ears
- (–) discharge from ears
- (–) H/O head injury

PAST MEDICAL HISTORY

- (+) H/O ruptured appendix, age 36, with IV antibiotics for 2 weeks
- (–) current medications
- (–) allergies

SOCIAL HISTORY

- Mechanical engineer
- Married, one son, age 16
- (+) "few beers a week"
- (–) recreational drug use
- (+) H/O syphilis, while in college

FAMILY HISTORY

- Mother—80 years old, severe osteoarthritis, diabetes
- Father died—lung cancer, age 70
- Brother—HT

PHYSICAL EXAMINATION—Include any significant pertinent positives and negatives

GENERAL

- Physical examination reveals a well-developed, obese, 55-year-old man appearing his stated age, holding his head, and complaining of severe dizziness

VITAL SIGNS

- BP 130/70
- Otherwise WNL

HEAD, EARS, EYES, NOSE, AND THROAT

- PERRL
- EOMs intact
- Discs clear with sharp disc margins; color WNL; vasculature WNL
- (–) discharge in external auditory canals
- TMs WNL
- Rinne—AC>BC bilaterally
- Weber—no lateralization

NEUROLOGICAL

- DTRs intact (biceps, triceps, patellar, Achilles—all 2+ bilaterally)
- Gait—patient refused because of extreme dizziness

DIFFERENTIAL DIAGNOSIS

In order of likelihood, write no more than five (5) differential diagnoses

1. Vestibular neuronitis
2. Ménière's disease
3. Labyrinthitis
4. Benign positional vertigo
5. Acoustic neuroma

DIAGNOSTIC WORKUP

Immediate plans, write no more than five (5) diagnostic studies

1. MRI/MRA of brain
2. CBC, electrolytes, glucose, BUN, creatinine, VDRL/RPR
3. Audiogram
4. Electronystagmography
5. ______________________________

CASE 12—Ms. Joy Devereaux

Ms. Joy Devereaux, a 55-year-old woman, presents to clinic complaining of difficulty in swallowing.

VITAL SIGNS

Temperature: 98.6° F	**Pulse:** 80 regular
Blood Pressure: 130/70	**Respiratory Rate:** 12 regular

EXAMINEE'S TASKS

In the next 15 minutes, you are to:

1) Take a focused history
2) Do a focused physical examination
3) Discuss your initial clinical impressions and workup plans with the patient
4) Write the Patient Note after leaving the room

Examinee's Data Gathering (DG) Checklists

HISTORY CHECKLIST

1. ______
2. ______
3. ______
4. ______
5. ______
6. ______
7. ______
8. ______
9. ______
10. ______
11. ______
12. ______
13. ______
14. ______
15. ______
16. ______
17. ______
18. ______
19. ______
20. ______
21. ______
22. ______
23. ______

PHYSICAL EXAMINATION CHECKLIST

1. ______
2. ______
3. ______
4. ______

5. ______________________________

6. ______________________________

Total DG Score ______ *Passing Score for DG is 20 points (70%)*

Examinee's Communication and Interpersonal Skills (CIS) Checklist

1. ______________________________
2. ______________________________
3. ______________________________
4. ______________________________
5. ______________________________
6. ______________________________
7. ______________________________
8. ______________________________
9. ______________________________
10. ______________________________
11. ______________________________
12. ______________________________
13. ______________________________
14. ______________________________
15. ______________________________
16. ______________________________
17. ______________________________
18. ______________________________
19. ______________________________
20. ______________________________

Total CIS Score ______ *Passing Score for CIS is 14 points (70%)*

123 Examinee's Spoken English Proficiency (SEP) Rating Scale

	Poor	Fair	Good	Very Good	Excellent
1. Ability of *patient* to understand *candidate*	1	2	3	4	5
2. Ability of *candidate* to understand *patient*	1	2	3	4	5
3. Candidate is articulate	1	2	3	4	5
4. Words are pronounced correctly	1	2	3	4	5
5. Range of vocabulary and sentence structure	1	2	3	4	5
6. Stress, rhythm, and intonation	1	2	3	4	5
7. Grammar	1	2	3	4	5
8. Repair strategies	1	2	3	4	5

Total SEP Score ______ *Passing Score for SEP is 28 points (70%)*

Examinee's Patient Note (PN)

HISTORY—Include any significant pertinent positives and negatives

PHYSICAL EXAMINATION—Include any significant pertinent positives and negatives

DIFFERENTIAL DIAGNOSIS

In order of likelihood, write no more than five (5) differential diagnoses

1.
2.
3.
4.
5.

DIAGNOSTIC WORKUP

Immediate plans, write no more than five (5) diagnostic studies

1.
2.
3.
4.
5.

Background Information for Standardized Patient

PATIENT BEHAVIOR
Agitated; crosses and uncrosses her legs frequently; puts her hand to her throat.

AFFECT
Unsettled; makes the doctor nervous as well.

PROVOCATIVE QUESTION(S) AND PLAUSIBLE ANSWER(S)
"Will I ever feel better again?"

"It's very hard to say at this point before we have all the information. As soon as I have the test results, I'll be in a better position to answer your question."

ADDITIONAL NOTES
The candidate will need to assess the appropriateness of counseling for quitting smoking *at this time*. Although this will be recommended for a long-term solution, at this initial evaluation the topic may be met with hostility. The candidate will need to evaluate how far to take this subject.

CHIEF COMPLAINT
"Difficulty in swallowing"

HISTORY OF PRESENT ILLNESS
Joy Devereaux is a 55-year-old woman who comes to clinic today complaining of difficulty in swallowing. For the past $2\frac{1}{2}$ months, she has had difficulty in swallowing. She says it feels like food gets stuck in her chest. It started with solid foods, but it has progressed so that now she has difficulty with liquids and even apple sauce. She does not have any pain except for the feeling of food getting stuck. She doesn't know of anything that makes it better or worse. She has also had a 15-pound weight loss in the past $2\frac{1}{2}$ months associated with loss of appetite. She is unaware of hoarseness, cough, hot/cold intolerance, fever, chills, vomiting, nausea, or diarrhea. She has never had anything like this in the past. There is no history of lye ingestion.

PAST MEDICAL HISTORY
For the past 10 years, she has a history of chronic heartburn for which she has been taking cimetidine.

MEDICATIONS
Cimetidine 200 mg two to three times daily
Aspirin

ALLERGIES
None

SOCIAL HISTORY
She is a cashier at the neighborhood produce store where she has worked for the past 17 years. She has smoked cigarettes, 2 packs per day, for the past 20 years. She also enjoys drinking vodka with cranberry juice, and she has been drinking about 6–8 ounces of alcohol nightly for the past 15 years. She doesn't use any other recreational drugs. She has never tried to cut down. She thinks that at some times others have been annoyed with her drinking. On occasion, about once or twice a year, she feels guilty about her drinking. She never has needed to start her day with alcohol; she drinks only in the evening.

FAMILY HISTORY
She is divorced for the past 4 years, and she has three children: a boy, age 22; a girl, age 20; and a boy, age 17. Her parents are both deceased. Her mother died of lung cancer at age 59, and her father died of liver cancer at age 64. She has no siblings.

SEXUAL HISTORY
She has not been sexually active for several years.

REVIEW OF SYSTEMS
Noncontributory

SP's Data Gathering (DG) Checklists

HISTORY CHECKLIST

1. For the past $2^1/_2$ months, I've had difficulty in swallowing.
2. It feels like food gets stuck in my chest.
3. It started with solid foods, but it has progressed so now I have difficulty even with liquids and apple sauce.
4. I do not have any pain except for the feeling of food getting stuck.
5. Nothing seems to make it better or worse.
6. I've lost 15 pounds in the past $2^1/_2$ months.
7. I don't seem to have an interest in food anymore.
8. I do not have hoarseness.
9. I don't have a cough.
10. I do not have hot or cold intolerance.
11. I do not have a fever or chills.
12. I don't have vomiting or nausea.
13. I don't have diarrhea.
14. I have never had anything like this before.
15. I've never ingested lye.
16. For the past 10 years, I've had chronic heartburn.
17. I take cimetidine for the heartburn—about 2–3 pills a day.
18. I have no allergies.
19. I smoke cigarettes, 2 packs per day for the past 20 years.
20. I enjoy drinking vodka with cranberry juice.
21. I have been drinking about 6–8 ounces of alcohol nightly for the past 15 years.
22. I do not use any other recreational drugs.
23. My father died of liver cancer at age 64.

PHYSICAL CHECKLIST

1. Evaluated throat by inspection for tonsillar enlargement
2. Evaluated thyroid by palpation—anterior and posterior
3. Evaluated for supraclavicular lymphadenopathy
4. Evaluated lung fields by auscultation
5. Evaluated abdomen by deep palpation (4 quadrants)
6. Evaluated liver by palpation

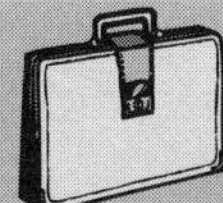

Examinee's Communication and Interpersonal Skills (CIS) Checklist

1. Knocked before entering
2. Opened interview by introducing self
3. Addressed patient using last name with introduction (e.g., Ms. Devereaux)
4. Appearance (e.g., clean and neat)
5. Allowed patient to express reason for seeking medical attention
6. Made comfortable eye contact
7. Did *not* use leading/biased questions (e.g., "You don't have…" or "You're not…")
8. Asked questions individually
9. Did *not* use the "Why" question
10. Concentrated and focused on patient's needs
11. Maintained comfortable and appropriate distance
12. Gave patient time to think and answer without interrupting
13. Used proper draping during physical exam
14. Did physical examination in an orderly manner
15. Summarized patient's condition (or asked patient to summarize)
16. Discussed diagnostic tests and/or next step in treatment in lay terms
17. Asked whether patient had other questions/concerns
18. Provided patient education/suggestions where appropriate
19. Did *not* give false assurances
20. Showed empathy

123 SP's Spoken English Proficiency (SEP) Rating Scale

	Poor	Fair	Good	Very Good	Excellent
1. Ability of *patient* to understand *candidate*	1	2	3	4	5
2. Ability of *candidate* to understand *patient*	1	2	3	4	5
3. Candidate is articulate	1	2	3	4	5
4. Words are pronounced correctly	1	2	3	4	5
5. Range of vocabulary and sentence structure	1	2	3	4	5
6. Stress, rhythm, and intonation	1	2	3	4	5
7. Grammar	1	2	3	4	5
8. Repair strategies	1	2	3	4	5

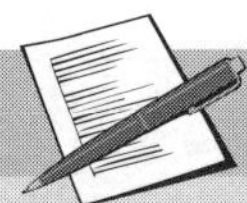

Example of a Satisfactory Patient Note (PN)

HISTORY—Include any significant pertinent positives and negatives

Ms. Joy Devereaux is a 55-year-old woman who comes for evaluation of difficulty in swallowing for the past 2½ months.

HISTORY OF PRESENT ILLNESS

- Food gets stuck in her chest
- Started with solid foods; now difficulty with liquids and even apple sauce
- (−) pain except for the feeling of food getting stuck
- Except for eating, nothing makes it better or worse
- (+) 15-pound weight loss in the past 2½ months associated with loss of appetite
- (−) hoarseness, cough, hot/cold intolerance, fever, chills, vomiting, nausea, or diarrhea
- (−) lye ingestion

PAST MEDICAL HISTORY

- (+) Chronic heartburn and takes cimetidine 2–3 × day
- (−) allergies

SOCIAL HISTORY

- Employed as cashier
- (+) 40 pack/year H/O smoking
- (+) Drinks vodka with cranberry juice; 6–8 ounces alcohol nightly for the past 15 years
- (−) tried to cut down
- (+/−) others annoyed at her drinking
- (+) sometimes feels guilty about her drinking
- (−) alcohol as eye-opener

FAMILY HISTORY

- Divorced for past 4 years
- 3 children: son, age 22; daughter, age 20; son, age 17
- Mother—died age 59 lung cancer
- Father—died age 64 liver cancer

SEXUAL HISTORY

(−) Sexually inactive for past several years

PHYSICAL EXAMINATION—Include any significant pertinent positives and negatives

GENERAL

- Physical examination reveals an ill-appearing, thin, 55-year-old woman appearing older than her stated age and complaining of difficulty swallowing.

VITAL SIGNS

- BP 130/70
- Otherwise WNL

HEAD, EARS, EYES, NOSE, AND THROAT

- (–) tonsillar enlargement
- (–) thyroid tenderness or masses by anterior and posterior palpation
- (–) supraclavicular or axillary adenopathy

CHEST

- Clear to P&A

HEART

- PMI 5th ICS-MCL
- S_1S_2 WNL
- (–) murmurs, gallops, or rubs

ABDOMEN

- (+) BS
- (–) tenderness
- (–) masses
- (–) hepatosplenomegaly

DIFFERENTIAL DIAGNOSIS

In order of likelihood, write no more than five (5) differential diagnoses

1. Esophageal carcinoma
2. Esophageal stricture
3. Achalasia
4. Gastric carcinoma
5. Chronic esophagitis

DIAGNOSTIC WORKUP

Immediate plans, write no more than five (5) diagnostic studies

1. Rectal exam and stool for FOBT
2. CBC, AST, ALT, bilirubin, alkaline phosphatase, albumin
3. Upper endoscopy and biopsy
4. Barium swallow
5. CT scan of the chest and abdomen

CASE 13—Mr. Tomas Sanchez

Mr. Tomas Sanchez, a 41-year-old man, presents to clinic complaining of abdominal pain and jaundice.

VITAL SIGNS

Temperature: 99.9° F	**Pulse:** 75 regular
Blood Pressure: 127/70	**Respiratory Rate:** 14 regular

EXAMINEE'S TASKS

In the next 15 minutes, you are to:

1. Take a focused history
2. Do a focused physical examination
3. Discuss your initial clinical impressions and workup plans with the patient
4. Write the Patient Note after leaving the room

Examinee's Data Gathering (DG) Checklists

HISTORY CHECKLIST

1. ______
2. ______
3. ______
4. ______
5. ______
6. ______
7. ______
8. ______
9. ______
10. ______
11. ______
12. ______
13. ______
14. ______
15. ______
16. ______
17. ______
18. ______
19. ______
20. ______
21. ______
22. ______
23. ______
24. ______

PHYSICAL EXAMINATION CHECKLIST

1. ______
2. ______
3. ______
4. ______

5. ____
6. ____
7. ____

Total DG Score ______ *Passing Score for DG is 22 points (70%)*

Examinee's Communication and Interpersonal Skills (CIS) Checklist

1. ____
2. ____
3. ____
4. ____
5. ____
6. ____
7. ____
8. ____
9. ____
10. ____
11. ____
12. ____
13. ____
14. ____
15. ____
16. ____
17. ____
18. ____
19. ____
20. ____

Total CIS Score ______ *Passing Score for CIS is 14 points (70%)*

123 Examinee's Spoken English Proficiency (SEP) Rating Scale

	Poor	Fair	Good	Very Good	Excellent
1. Ability of *patient* to understand *candidate*	1	2	3	4	5
2. Ability of *candidate* to understand *patient*	1	2	3	4	5
3. Candidate is articulate	1	2	3	4	5
4. Words are pronounced correctly	1	2	3	4	5
5. Range of vocabulary and sentence structure	1	2	3	4	5
6. Stress, rhythm, and intonation	1	2	3	4	5
7. Grammar	1	2	3	4	5
8. Repair strategies	1	2	3	4	5

Total SEP Score ______ *Passing Score for SEP is 28 points (70%)*

Examinee's Patient Note (PN)

HISTORY—Include any significant pertinent positives and negatives

PHYSICAL EXAMINATION—Include any significant pertinent positives and negatives

DIFFERENTIAL DIAGNOSIS

In order of likelihood, write no more than five (5) differential diagnoses

1.
2.
3.
4.
5.

DIAGNOSTIC WORKUP

Immediate plans, write no more than five (5) diagnostic studies

1.
2.
3.
4.
5.

Background Information for Standardized Patient

PATIENT BEHAVIOR

Fake smile; wouldn't be here except for the pain.

AFFECT

Nervous; doesn't want to face the inevitable questions about alcohol.

PROVOCATIVE QUESTION(S) AND PLAUSIBLE ANSWER(S)

"Are you going to cure me, doc?

"We are going to do everything we can to make you better, but we first need to do some tests to find out what's wrong with you."

ADDITIONAL NOTES

Yellow eyes

If you suspect someone might be an alcoholic and are going to start the CAGE questions, be careful how you approach the patient. You may be forcing them to look at aspects of their life that they are not ready to face. The manner in which they answer the questions may be just as telling as the answers themselves.

CHIEF COMPLAINT

"I've got stomach pain and my eyes are yellow."

HISTORY OF PRESENT ILLNESS

Tomas Sanchez is a 41-year-old man who came to clinic today because he has had abdominal pain for the past 4 days, and his friend noted this morning that his eyes had turned yellow. The pain is like a gnawing ache and is located below his right rib case. It's about a 5 or 6 out of 10 in severity. Nothing seems to make it better or worse. The pain is there all the time. The pain is only in his abdomen and is not felt in any other part of his body. He's also been having nausea and has vomited several times in the past 24 hours.

He has also noticed that since yesterday, his urine is really dark, and his bowel movements are really light, like clay.

Over the past month, he has lost about 10 pounds. He was not trying to lose weight, but nothing tastes good to him.

He has noticed that he does feel warm but has not taken his temperature. He does not have chills. He does not have any pain in his joints or itching.

PAST MEDICAL HISTORY

About 14 months ago, he vomited blood and was taken to the hospital where he received a transfusion of 2 units of blood.

MEDICATIONS

None

ALLERGIES

None

SOCIAL HISTORY

He is a house painter. He's had a live-in girlfriend for 3 years, and they have 2 children.

He's been a heavy drinker for the past 10–12 years and enjoys drinking a six-pack of beer and rum daily. Six days before coming to clinic, his best friend got engaged, and a group of guys went out drinking. He got really drunk and had to stay in bed for almost 24 hours.

He enjoys smoking pot when it's available. He has been smoking about 1½ packs of cigarettes a day for the past 15 years.

FAMILY HISTORY

His mother is 62 years old and has diabetes. His father died of cirrhosis at age 56. He was an alcoholic. His only brother died of AIDS at age 39 several years ago.

SEXUAL HISTORY

He has not been sexually active for the past 10 days. He feels tired and weak all the time.

REVIEW OF SYSTEMS

Noncontributory

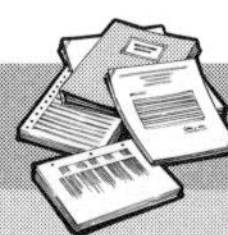

SP's Data Gathering (DG) Checklists

HISTORY CHECKLIST

1. I came to clinic today because I've got stomach pain and my eyes are yellow.
2. I've had the pain for the past 4 days.
3. My friend noted this morning that my eyes are yellow.
4. The pain is like a gnawing ache.
5. The pain is located below my right rib cage.
6. The pain is about a 5 or 6 out of 10 in severity.
7. Nothing seems to make the pain better or worse.
8. The pain is there all the time.
9. The pain is only in my stomach; I don't feel it in any other part of my body.
10. I've been having nausea for the past 24 hours.
11. I vomited several times in the past 24 hours.
12. I've been a heavy drinker for the past 10–12 years.
13. I drink a six-pack of beer and rum daily.
14. Six days before coming to clinic, I got really drunk.
15. Since yesterday, my urine is really dark.
16. My bowel movements are really light—like clay—since yesterday.
17. I have lost about 10 pounds in the past month.
18. Nothing tastes good to me.
19. I feel warm, but I have not taken my temperature.
20. I do not have chills.
21. I do not have any pain in my joints.
22. I do not have any itching.
23. Fourteen months ago, I received a transfusion of 2 units of blood.
24. I have no allergies.

PHYSICAL CHECKLIST

1. Took blood pressure
2. Performed light palpation of the abdomen in all 4 quadrants *after* auscultation
3. Performed deep palpation of the abdomen in all 4 quadrants
4. Percussed abdomen in all 4 quadrants
5. Evaluated liver size
6. Evaluated spleen size
7. Evaluate abdomen for ascites

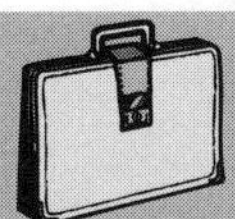

SP's Communication and Interpersonal Skills (CIS) Checklist

1. Knocked before entering
2. Opened interview by introducing self
3. Addressed patient using last name with introduction (e.g., Mr. Sanchez)
4. Appearance (e.g., clean and neat)
5. Allowed patient to express reason for seeking medical attention
6. Made comfortable eye contact
7. Did *not* use leading/biased questions (e.g., "You don't have…" or "You're not…")
8. Asked questions individually
9. Did *not* use the "Why" question
10. Concentrated and focused on patient's needs
11. Maintained comfortable and appropriate distance
12. Gave patient time to think and answer without interrupting
13. Used proper draping during physical exam
14. Did physical examination in an orderly manner
15. Summarized patient's condition (or asked patient to summarize)
16. Discussed diagnostic tests and/or next step in treatment in lay terms
17. Asked whether patient had other questions/concerns
18. Provided patient education/suggestions where appropriate
19. Did *not* give false assurances
20. Showed empathy

123 SP's Spoken English Proficiency (SEP) Rating Scale

	Poor	Fair	Good	Very Good	Excellent
1. Ability of *patient* to understand *candidate*	1	2	3	4	5
2. Ability of *candidate* to understand *patient*	1	2	3	4	5
3. Candidate is articulate	1	2	3	4	5
4. Words are pronounced correctly	1	2	3	4	5
5. Range of vocabulary and sentence structure	1	2	3	4	5
6. Stress, rhythm, and intonation	1	2	3	4	5
7. Grammar	1	2	3	4	5
8. Repair strategies	1	2	3	4	5

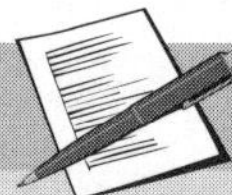

Example of a Satisfactory Patient Note (PN)

HISTORY—Include any significant pertinent positives and negatives

Mr. Tomas Sanchez is a 41-year-old chronic alcoholic who presents with the chief complaint of "stomach pain and my eyes are yellow."

HISTORY OF PRESENT ILLNESS

- Abdominal pain for the past 4 days
- Scleral icterus since this morning
- Pain is gnawing ache, located below his right rib cage, about a 5 or 6/10 in severity
- Nothing seems to make the pain better or worse; no radiation of pain
- (+) nausea for the past 24 hours.
- (+) vomiting in the past 24 hours
- Heavy drinker for the past 10–12 years; drinks a six-pack of beer and rum daily
- Six days before coming to clinic, got really drunk
- Urine very dark; bowel movements clay colored since yesterday
- (+) 10-pound weight loss in the past month
- No appetite in past month
- Feels warm but has not taken temperature
- (–) chills, arthralgias, pruritus

PAST MEDICAL HISTORY

- (+) Transfusion of 2 units of blood 14 months ago
- (–) Allergies

SOCIAL HISTORY

- House painter
- Lives with girlfriend and 2 children
- (+) smokes pot when available
- (+) 1½ ppd of cigarettes for the past 15 years

FAMILY HISTORY

- Mother—62 years old, diabetes
- Father died—cirrhosis, age 56; alcoholic
- Brother died—AIDS, age 39

PHYSICAL EXAMINATION—Include any significant pertinent positives and negatives

GENERAL

- Physical examination reveals a sickly appearing, 41-year-old man, appearing older than his stated age and complaining of RUQ pain

VITAL SIGNS

- BP 125/70
- Otherwise WNL

ABDOMEN

- Slightly distended
- (+) bowel sounds
- (+) mild tenderness RUQ
- (−) masses
- Liver span 10 cm, MCL
- (−) spleen
- (−) ascites

DIFFERENTIAL DIAGNOSIS

In order of likelihood, write no more than five (5) differential diagnoses

1. Acute viral hepatitis
2. Acute alcoholic hepatitis
3. Acute cholecystitis
4. Acute pancreatitis
5. Hepatocellular carcinoma

DIAGNOSTIC WORKUP

Immediate plans, write no more than five (5) diagnostic studies

1. Rectal exam and stool for FOBT
2. CBC, amylase, lipase, AST, ALT, alkaline phosphatase, BUN, creatinine, Ca^{2+}, GGT
3. Viral hepatitis serologies (HCV antigen, anti-HCV, HBsAg, HBsAb, HBcAb)
4. Abdominal ultrasonogram
5. U/A

CASE 14—Ms. Wendy Blalock

Ms. Wendy Blalock, a 55-year-old woman, presents to clinic complaining of vaginal bleeding.

VITAL SIGNS

Temperature: 98.6° F	**Pulse:** 80 regular
Blood Pressure: 130/70	**Respiratory Rate:** 12 regular

EXAMINEE'S TASKS

In the next 15 minutes, you are to:

1. Take a focused history
2. Do a focused physical examination
3. Discuss your initial clinical impressions and workup plans with the patient
4. Write the Patient Note after leaving the room

Examinee's Data Gathering (DG) Checklists

HISTORY CHECKLIST

1. ____
2. ____
3. ____
4. ____
5. ____
6. ____
7. ____
8. ____
9. ____
10. ____
11. ____
12. ____
13. ____
14. ____
15. ____
16. ____
17. ____
18. ____
19. ____
20. ____
21. ____

PHYSICAL EXAMINATION CHECKLIST

1. ____
2. ____
3. ____
4. ____
5. ____

6. ____
7. ____

Total DG Score ______ *Passing Score for DG is 20 points (70%)*

Examinee's Communication and Interpersonal Skills (CIS) Checklist

1. ____
2. ____
3. ____
4. ____
5. ____
6. ____
7. ____
8. ____
9. ____
10. ____
11. ____
12. ____
13. ____
14. ____
15. ____
16. ____
17. ____
18. ____
19. ____
20. ____

Total CIS Score ______ *Passing Score for CIS is 14 points (70%)*

123 Examinee's Spoken English Proficiency (SEP) Rating Scale

	Poor	Fair	Good	Very Good	Excellent
1. Ability of *patient* to understand *candidate*	1	2	3	4	5
2. Ability of *candidate* to understand *patient*	1	2	3	4	5
3. Candidate is articulate	1	2	3	4	5
4. Words are pronounced correctly	1	2	3	4	5
5. Range of vocabulary and sentence structure	1	2	3	4	5
6. Stress, rhythm, and intonation	1	2	3	4	5
7. Grammar	1	2	3	4	5
8. Repair strategies	1	2	3	4	5

Total SEP Score ______ *Passing Score for SEP is 28 points (70%)*

Examinee's Patient Note (PN)

HISTORY—Include any significant pertinent positives and negatives

PHYSICAL EXAMINATION— Include any significant pertinent positives and negatives

DIFFERENTIAL DIAGNOSIS

In order of likelihood, write no more than five (5) differential diagnoses

1.
2.
3.
4.
5.

DIAGNOSTIC WORKUP

Immediate plans, write no more than five (5) diagnostic studies

1.
2.
3.
4.
5.

Background Information for Standardized Patient

PATIENT BEHAVIOR

Pursed lips; perhaps nail biting or some other small nervous habit is displayed.

AFFECT

Controlled panic

PROVOCATIVE QUESTION(S) AND PLAUSIBLE ANSWER(S)

"I'm worried that there is something really wrong with me. Why would I be bleeding if I am already postmenopausal?"

"I can certainly understand your concern, and it is good that you came in to see me today. We need to further explore your situation, and do some tests before we will know anything definitive. Rest assured, you are in good hands."

CHIEF COMPLAINT

"Vaginal bleeding"

HISTORY OF PRESENT ILLNESS

Wendy Blalock is a 55-year-old woman who presents to clinic for evaluation of vaginal bleeding. She started having intermittent vaginal spotting about a month ago. Yesterday, she noted more vaginal bleeding. This morning she passed a blood clot, so she came in for evaluation. Her last menstrual period was 6 years ago. There is no associated vaginal discharge, pain, or urinary symptoms. She denies any vaginal or abdominal injury. She has no history of easy bruisability or blood problem. She saw her gynecologist about 6 months ago, and all seemed fine. A Pap smear was normal.

PAST MEDICAL HISTORY

She has a history of breast cancer (estrogen-receptor positive) treated with a modified radical left mastectomy, chemotherapy, and radiotherapy 4 years ago. She was started on tamoxifen 3 years ago. She has no history of nausea or hot flashes. Her last mammogram was 4 months ago, and it was normal. She has not been tested for BRCA. She has a history of high blood pressure, which is well controlled on medications.

MEDICATIONS

Lisinopril 20 mg daily
Tamoxifen 20 mg daily
Fosamax 70 mg weekly (every Sunday)

ALLERGIES
None

SOCIAL HISTORY
She is a high school English teacher. She is married with four children, ranging in age from 18 to 24. She has three sons and one daughter, age 20. She never smoked. She enjoys a glass of wine when she socializes with friends on the weekend. She has never used any other recreational drugs.

FAMILY HISTORY
Her mother had breast cancer at age 61; she is now 76 and is doing well. Her father has peptic ulcer disease with recurrent ulcers and Ménière's disease.

SEXUAL HISTORY
She is sexually active with only her husband of 25 years, although her sex drive has been reduced over the past 3–4 months. She now has sexual relations about once or twice a month.

REVIEW OF SYSTEMS
Noncontributory

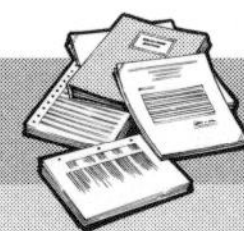

SP's Data Gathering (DG) Checklists

HISTORY CHECKLIST

1. I've got vaginal bleeding.
2. It started with intermittent vaginal spotting about a month ago.
3. Yesterday, there was more vaginal bleeding, and this morning there was a blood clot.
4. My last menstrual period was 6 years ago.
5. I've never had any vaginal discharge.
6. I don't have vaginal pain.
7. I don't have any urinary symptoms.
8. I have never had any vaginal or abdominal injury.
9. I haven't noticed any easy bruising.
10. I don't have any bleeding problem.
11. I saw my gynecologist about 6 months ago, and all seemed fine.
12. I had a Pap smear which was normal about 6 months ago.
13. I had breast cancer (estrogen-receptor positive) 4 years ago.
14. I had a modified radical left mastectomy, chemotherapy, and radiotherapy.
15. I was started on tamoxifen 3 years ago.
16. I have no history of nausea or hot flashes.
17. My last mammogram was 4 months ago, and it was normal.
18. I have never been tested for BRCA.
19. I've had high blood pressure, which has been well-controlled with medications for many years.
20. My mother had breast cancer at age 61; she is now 76 and is doing well.
21. I have one daughter, age 20.

PHYSICAL CHECKLIST

1. Took blood pressure
2. Evaluated for orthostatic hypotension
3. Performed light palpation of the abdomen in all 4 quadrants *after* auscultation
4. Performed deep palpation of the abdomen in all 4 quadrants
5. Percussed abdomen in all 4 quadrants
7. Evaluated liver by palpation

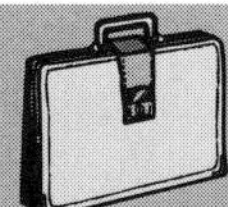

SP's Communication and Interpersonal Skills (CIS) Checklist

1. Knocked before entering
2. Opened interview by introducing self
3. Addressed patient using last name with introduction (e.g., Ms. Blalock)
4. Appearance (e.g., clean and neat)
5. Allowed patient to express reason for seeking medical attention
6. Made comfortable eye contact
7. Did *not* use leading/biased questions (e.g., "You don't have…" or "You're not…")
8. Asked questions individually
9. Did *not* use the "Why" question
10. Concentrated and focused on patient's needs
11. Maintained comfortable and appropriate distance
12. Gave patient time to think and answer without interrupting
13. Used proper draping during physical exam
14. Did physical examination in an orderly manner
15. Summarized patient's condition (or asked patient to summarize)
16. Discussed diagnostic tests and/or next step in treatment in lay terms
17. Asked whether patient had other questions/concerns
18. Provided patient education/suggestions where appropriate
19. Did *not* give false assurances
20. Showed empathy

123 SP's Spoken English Proficiency (SEP) Rating Scale

	Poor	Fair	Good	Very Good	Excellent
1. Ability of *patient* to understand *candidate*	1	2	3	4	5
2. Ability of *candidate* to understand *patient*	1	2	3	4	5
3. Candidate is articulate	1	2	3	4	5
4. Words are pronounced correctly	1	2	3	4	5
5. Range of vocabulary and sentence structure	1	2	3	4	5
6. Stress, rhythm, and intonation	1	2	3	4	5
7. Grammar	1	2	3	4	5
8. Repair strategies	1	2	3	4	5

Example of a Satisfactory Patient Note (PN)

HISTORY—Include any significant pertinent positives and negatives

Ms. Wendy Blalock is a 55-year-old woman, S/P breast cancer, now on tamoxifen, who presents with vaginal bleeding

HISTORY OF PRESENT ILLNESS

- Intermittent vaginal spotting started 1 month ago
- More bleeding yesterday and this AM a clot
- LMP—6 years ago
- (−) vaginal discharge, pain, or urinary symptoms
- (−) H/O vaginal trauma
- (−) easy bruisability or blood problems
- Saw gynecologist 6 months ago—all normal including Pap smear

PAST MEDICAL HISTORY

- (+) H/O estrogen receptor positive breast cancer 4 years ago
- Treated with modified radical left mastectomy, chemotherapy, and radiotherapy
- Tamoxifen therapy for past 3 years
- (−) nausea or hot flashes
- Last mammogram 4 months ago—normal
- Never tested for BRCA mutation
- (+) H/O HT—on medications for years
- medications
  Lisinopril 20 mg daily
  Tamoxifen 20 mg daily
  Fosamax 70 mg weekly (every Sunday)
- (−) allergies

SOCIAL HISTORY

- High school English teacher
- Married, 4 children: 3 sons and 1 daughter age 20
- (+) social drinker
- (−) H/O smoking
- (−) recreational drug use

FAMILY HISTORY

- Mother—76 years old, breast cancer at age 61
- Father—77 years old, peptic ulcer disease and Ménière's disease

SEXUAL HISTORY

- Sexually active with only her husband of 25 years
- Reduced sex drive for past 3–4 months

PHYSICAL EXAMINATION—Include any significant pertinent positives and negatives

GENERAL

- Physical examination reveals a well-developed, slightly obese, 54-year-old woman appearing her stated age and complaining of vaginal bleeding.

VITAL SIGNS

- BP 130/70
- (–) orthostatic hypotension
- Otherwise WNL

ABDOMEN

- (+) BS
- (–) tenderness elicited
- (–) masses palpated
- (–) hepatosplenomegaly

DIFFERENTIAL DIAGNOSIS

In order of likelihood, write no more than five (5) differential diagnoses

1. Endometrial carcinoma
2. Cervical carcinoma
3. Atrophic endometrium
4. Endometrial polyps
5. Drug-induced (tamoxifen) endometrial hyperplasia

DIAGNOSTIC WORKUP

Immediate plans, write no more than five (5) diagnostic studies

1. Pelvic exam and Pap smear
2. Endometrial biopsy
3. Ultrasound of pelvis
4. Endometrial curettage
5. Colposcopy

CASE 15—Jesse Prince

Mrs. Prince has called your office about her 2½-year-old son, Jesse. She wants to speak to you about her son who awoke coughing last night. Please call Mrs. Prince back at (999) 123-4567.

EXAMINEE'S TASKS

In the next 15 minutes, you are to:

1. Take a focused history from the mother over the telephone
2. Discuss your initial clinical impressions and workup plans with Mrs. Prince
3. Write the Patient Note after leaving the room

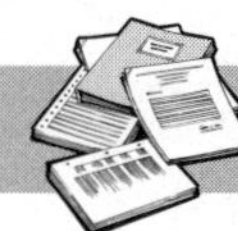

Examinee's Data Gathering (DG) Checklists

HISTORY CHECKLIST

1. ______
2. ______
3. ______
4. ______
5. ______
6. ______
7. ______
8. ______
9. ______
10. ______
11. ______
12. ______
13. ______
14. ______
15. ______
16. ______
17. ______
18. ______
19. ______
20. ______
21. ______
22. ______

Total DG Score ______ *Passing Score for DG is 15 points (70%)*

Examinee's Communication and Interpersonal Skills (CIS) Checklist

1. ______
2. ______
3. ______
4. ______
5. ______
6. ______
7. ______
8. ______
9. ______
10. ______
11. ______
12. ______
13. ______
14. ______

Total CIS Score ______ *Passing Score for CIS is 10 points (70%)*

123 Examinee's Spoken English Proficiency (SEP) Rating Scale

	Poor	Fair	Good	Very Good	Excellent
1. Ability of *patient* to understand *candidate*	1	2	3	4	5
2. Ability of *candidate* to understand *patient*	1	2	3	4	5
3. Candidate is articulate	1	2	3	4	5
4. Words are pronounced correctly	1	2	3	4	5
5. Range of vocabulary and sentence structure	1	2	3	4	5
6. Stress, rhythm, and intonation	1	2	3	4	5
7. Grammar	1	2	3	4	5
8. Repair strategies	1	2	3	4	5

Total SEP Score _____ *Passing Score for SEP is 28 points (70%)*

Examinee's Patient Note (PN)

HISTORY— Include any significant pertinent positives and negatives

PHYSICAL EXAMINATION—Include any significant pertinent positives and negatives

DIFFERENTIAL DIAGNOSIS

In order of likelihood, write no more than five (5) differential diagnoses

1.
2.
3.
4.
5.

DIAGNOSTIC WORKUP

Immediate plans, write no more than five (5) diagnostic studies

1.
2.
3.
4.
5.

Background Information for Standardized Patient

PATIENT BEHAVIOR

Agitated; concerned about her son

AFFECT

Nice; concerned

PROVOCATIVE QUESTION(S) AND PLAUSIBLE ANSWER(S)

"What do you think is wrong with Jesse?"

"I think it is very important to bring Jesse in immediately so we can take a look at him. Then, we will be better able to answer your question."

CHIEF COMPLAINT

"My son is coughing a lot."

HISTORY OF PRESENT ILLNESS

Mrs. Prince has just called your office wanting to speak to you about her son Jesse who awoke last night with a coughing fit.

Jesse is 2½ years old and has been in good health. He weighs 29 pounds, is 34 inches tall, and is in the middle of all his growth curves. Over the past 3–4 days, Jesse has had a runny nose and cough. He awoke last night at 2 AM with a severe cough. He was breathing very fast and couldn't talk. Mrs. Prince also noticed that he was "burning up" last night, and she gave him some Tylenol Cold. He also vomited about three times and brought up clear, yellowish fluid. She thought that the vomiting might be a result of his coughing spell. He didn't bring up any sputum. When he coughed, she thought that she heard him wheeze, and she was up all night with Jesse. He's a little better now, but he's not himself. His breathing is better, but Mrs. Prince feels that there is something wrong: "Do the coughs seem to hurt him?"

Jesse has been eating and drinking less for the past week, and he looks sick and doesn't want to play. He also wants to be held more. He was last seen in the pediatrician's office 2 months ago and all seemed fine.

He doesn't snore or mouth breathe. There is no history of weight loss.

His 3-year-old cousin visited with Jesse last weekend, and he had a bad cold. Mrs. Prince asks, "Maybe Jesse caught it?"

He ate some peanuts about 2 weeks ago and started coughing. Mrs. Prince asks, "Could he have a peanut allergy?"

PAST MEDICAL HISTORY

All of Jesse's developmental milestones are normal. He is up-to-date with his immunizations. Mrs. Prince's pregnancy with Jesse was uneventful, and he was delivered vaginally. When Jesse was $1\frac{1}{2}$ years old, she was told that Jesse had a heart murmur; it was not evaluated. Jesse is her only child.

Jesse had one ear infection when he was 14 months old. He has had a few colds. He has never had pneumonia. There is no previous history of wheezing. There is no history of eczema.

MEDICATIONS

None

ALLERGIES

None. Mrs. Prince has not changed the detergent she uses to wash his clothes. Shes uses the same cleaning solutions that she has always used.

SOCIAL HISTORY

No one smokes in the house.

FAMILY HISTORY

Mrs. Prince works as a housekeeper for an older man Mr. Joshua White. During the day, her mother takes care of Jesse. Her mother was recently diagnosed with tuberculosis and is now on treatment with INH. Mrs. Prince is concerned about her job if she needs to take Jesse to the hospital or if her mother can't take care of Jesse. Mrs. Prince has never missed a day taking care of Mr. White. Mrs. Prince had asthma as a child.

SEXUAL HISTORY

NA

REVIEW OF SYSTEMS

Mrs. Prince states that she has had some construction work done in the past month in her apartment.

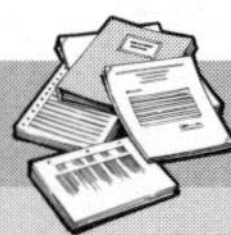

SP's Data Gathering (DG) Checklists

HISTORY CHECKLIST

1. My son Jesse awoke last light at 2 AM with a coughing fit.
2. He was breathing very fast and couldn't talk.
3. He was "burning up" last night with fever.
4. I gave him some Tylenol Cold.
5. He vomited about three times and brought up clear, yellowish fluid.
6. He didn't bring up any sputum.
7. When he coughed last night, I thought that he was wheezing,
8. Over the past 3–4 days, he's had a runny nose and cough.
9. Jesse has been eating and drinking less for the past week.
10. He was last seen in the pediatrician's office 2 months ago and all seemed fine.
11. He doesn't snore.
12. He hasn't lost any weight.
13. He ate some peanuts about 2 weeks ago and started coughing.
14. Jesse has been previously in good health.
15. He weighs 29 pounds and is 34 inches tall.
16. My pregnancy with Jesse was uneventful, and he was delivered vaginally.
17. When Jesse was 1½ years old, I was told that he had a heart murmur.
18. He has never had pneumonia.
19. There is no prior history of wheezing.
20. My mother was recently diagnosed with tuberculosis and is now on treatment with INH.
21. I had asthma as a child.
22. We have had some construction work done in the past month in our apartment.

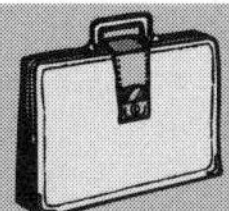

SP's Communication and Interpersonal Skills (CIS) Checklist

1. Opened interview by introducing self
2. Addressed patient using last name with introduction (e.g., Mrs. Prince)
3. Allowed patient to express reason for seeking medical attention
4. Did *not* use leading/biased questions (e.g., "You don't have…" or "You're not…")
5. Asked questions individually
6. Did *not* use the "Why" question
7. Concentrated and focused on patient's needs
8. Gave patient time to think and answer without interrupting
9. Summarized patient's condition (or asked patient to summarize)
10. Discussed diagnostic tests and/or next step in treatment in lay terms
11. Asked whether patient had other questions/concerns
12. Provided patient education/suggestions where appropriate
13. Did *not* give false assurances
14. Showed empathy

123 SP's Spoken English Proficiency (SEP) Rating Scale

	Poor	Fair	Good	Very Good	Excellent
1. Ability of *patient* to understand *candidate*	1	2	3	4	5
2. Ability of *candidate* to understand *patient*	1	2	3	4	5
3. Candidate is articulate	1	2	3	4	5
4. Words are pronounced correctly	1	2	3	4	5
5. Range of vocabulary and sentence structure	1	2	3	4	5
6. Stress, rhythm, and intonation	1	2	3	4	5
7. Grammar	1	2	3	4	5
8. Repair strategies	1	2	3	4	5

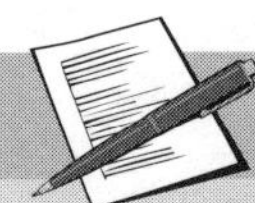

Example of a Satisfactory Patient Note (PN)

HISTORY—Include any significant pertinent positives and negatives

Jesse Prince is a 2½-year-old male whose mother has just called our office complaining that he was awakened last night with a coughing fit and requesting that we call her back.

HISTORY OF PRESENT ILLNESS

Jesse has been in good health. He awoke last night with a coughing fit. Over the past 3–4 days, Jesse had a runny nose and cough. His mother states that he was breathing very fast, couldn't talk, and was "burning up" last night; she gave him some Tylenol Cold. He also vomited about three times and brought up clear, yellowish fluid. She denies any sputum production. Mrs. Prince did mention that she thought she heard him wheeze. Mrs. Prince describes that Jesse has been eating and drinking less for the past week and looks sick and doesn't want to play. He also wants to be held more. There is no history of snoring, mouth breathing, or weight loss. Mrs. Prince also related that about 2 weeks ago he ate some peanuts and started coughing.

PAST MEDICAL HISTORY

Jesse was last seen in the pediatrician's office 2 months ago, and all seemed fine. He weighs 29 pounds, is 34 inches tall, and is in the middle of all his growth curves.

Jesse is up-to-date with his immunizations. Mrs. Prince's pregnancy with Jesse was uneventful, and he was delivered vaginally. When Jesse was 1½ years old, she was told that he had a heart murmur; it was not evaluated. Jesse is her only child. Jesse had one ear infection when he was 14 months old. He has had a few colds. He has never had pneumonia. There is no previous history of wheezing. There is no history of eczema.

He is not taking any medications. He has no known allergies. Mrs. Prince has not changed the detergent she uses to wash his clothes. She uses the same cleaning solutions that she has always used.

SOCIAL HISTORY

No one smokes in the house. Otherwise noncontributory.

FAMILY HISTORY

Mrs. Prince works as a housekeeper for an older man. During the day, her mother takes cares of Jesse. Her mother was recently diagnosed with tuberculosis and is now on treatment with INH.

Mrs. Prince had asthma as a child.

SUMMARY

I advised Mrs. Prince to bring Jesse in immediately to the ER. Although she was initially somewhat reluctant, I was able to convince her of the importance of the visit.

DIFFERENTIAL DIAGNOSIS

In order of likelihood, write no more than five (5) differential diagnoses

1. Asthma (viral induced)
2. Pneumonia
3. Tuberculosis
4. Foreign body aspiration
5. Congestive heart failure

DIAGNOSTIC WORKUP

Immediate plans, write no more than five (5) diagnostic studies

1. Chest x-ray—decubitus both sides
2. CBC, ESR
3. PPD
4. Spirometry
5. ______________________________

CASE 16—Ms. Betty Balcomb

Ms. Betty Balcomb, a 65-year-old woman, presents to clinic complaining of shortness of breath.

VITAL SIGNS

Temperature: 98.6° F	**Pulse:** 90 regular
Blood Pressure: 160/85	**Respiratory Rate:** 16 regular

EXAMINEE'S TASKS

In the next 15 minutes, you are to:

1. Take a focused history
2. Do a focused physical examination
3. Discuss your initial clinical impressions and workup plans with the patient
4. Write the Patient Note after leaving the room

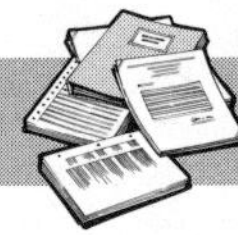

Examinee's Data Gathering (DG) Checklists

HISTORY CHECKLIST

1. ____________________
2. ____________________
3. ____________________
4. ____________________
5. ____________________
6. ____________________
7. ____________________
8. ____________________
9. ____________________
10. ____________________
11. ____________________
12. ____________________
13. ____________________
14. ____________________
15. ____________________
16. ____________________
17. ____________________
18. ____________________
19. ____________________
20. ____________________
21. ____________________

PHYSICAL EXAMINATION CHECKLIST

1. ____________________
2. ____________________
3. ____________________
4. ____________________
5. ____________________
6. ____________________

7. ____

8. ____

9. ____

10. ____

Total DG Score ______ *Passing Score for DG is 22 points (70%)*

Examinee's Communication and Interpersonal Skills (CIS) Checklist

1. ____
2. ____
3. ____
4. ____
5. ____
6. ____
7. ____
8. ____
9. ____
10. ____
11. ____
12. ____
13. ____
14. ____
15. ____
16. ____
17. ____
18. ____
19. ____
20. ____

Total CIS Score ______ *Passing Score for CIS is 14 points (70%)*

Examinee's Spoken English Proficiency (SEP) Rating Scale

	Poor	Fair	Good	Very Good	Excellent
1. Ability of *patient* to understand *candidate*	1	2	3	4	5
2. Ability of *candidate* to understand *patient*	1	2	3	4	5
3. Candidate is articulate	1	2	3	4	5
4. Words are pronounced correctly	1	2	3	4	5
5. Range of vocabulary and sentence structure	1	2	3	4	5
6. Stress, rhythm, and intonation	1	2	3	4	5
7. Grammar	1	2	3	4	5
8. Repair strategies	1	2	3	4	5

Total SEP Score _____ *Passing Score for SEP is 28 points (70%)*

Examinee's Patient Note (PN)

HISTORY—Include any significant pertinent positives and negatives

PHYSICAL EXAMINATION—Include any significant pertinent positives and negatives

DIFFERENTIAL DIAGNOSIS

In order of likelihood, write no more than five (5) differential diagnoses

1.
2.
3.
4.
5.

DIAGNOSTIC WORKUP

Immediate plans, write no more than five (5) diagnostic studies

1.
2.
3.
4.
5.

Background Information for Standardized Patient

PATIENT BEHAVIOR

Doesn't move around much; sighs; seems to be trying to catch her breath just sitting in the chair.

AFFECT

Sad; unsettled; worried

PROVOCATIVE QUESTION(S) AND PLAUSIBLE ANSWER(S)

"Am I going to have another heart attack?"

"It's good that you came in for evaluation now so we can take good care of you. At the present time, it doesn't appear that you are having another heart attack, but we need to do some tests."

ADDITIONAL NOTES

Although obviously it would be prudent to counsel this patient to quit smoking, the worrisome and worsening issues with her shortness of breath predominate. If in the limited time you spend with this patient you can at least touch upon her smoking, fine. But the majority of your time needs to address her worsening heart condition. Once you deal with that, the important issue of quitting smoking will come into play.

CHIEF COMPLAINT

"Shortness of breath"

HISTORY OF PRESENT ILLNESS

Betty Balcomb is a 65-year-old woman who is coming to clinic today for evaluation of worsening shortness of breath over the past 3 months. She now notices that she has shortness of breath after walking less than one level block. She remembers that only 3 months ago she could walk about 3–4 level blocks without becoming short of breath. She has also awakened from sleep with shortness of breath in the past few days, and about a week ago, she developed a cough at night with pink frothy sputum. She is aware that her shortness of breath is definitely worse when lying down and gets better when she sits up. She also needs to sleep on three pillows; 3 months ago she needed only one pillow. Over the past 2 months, she has put on about 10 pounds and has had significant swelling in her legs. Her appetite is also down.

She has not had recent chest pain, nausea, vomiting, or sweating.

PAST MEDICAL HISTORY

She had a heart attack 5 years ago and was hospitalized for 7 days. She has had high blood pressure for 25 years and high cholesterol for 15 years.

MEDICATIONS

Digoxin 0.25 mg daily
Hydrochlorothiazide 50 mg daily
Atenolol 50 mg daily
Simvastatin 20 mg daily
Aspirin daily

ALLERGIES

None

SOCIAL HISTORY

She is a retired librarian. She is married and has two sons, ages 39 and 41. She smokes 1½ packs per day for the past 35 years. She has tried to cut down, especially after her heart attack, but she has been unsuccessful in stopping to smoke.

FAMILY HISTORY

Her parents are deceased. Her mother died at age 85 of old age. Her father died of a stroke at age 74. Her only sister died 2 years ago of multiple myeloma at age 63.

SEXUAL HISTORY

She is married, but she has not been sexually active for some time. She just has no interest.

REVIEW OF SYSTEMS

Noncontributory

SP's Data Gathering (DG) Checklists

HISTORY CHECKLIST

1. My shortness of breath has been getting worse over the past 3 months.
2. I now get short of breath after walking less than 1 level block.
3. Three months ago I could walk about 3 to 4 level blocks without becoming short of breath.
4. I awaken from sleep with shortness of breath.
5. About a week ago, I developed a cough at night with pink frothy sputum.
6. The shortness of breath is definitely worse when lying down.
7. The shortness of breath gets better when I sit up.
8. I need to sleep on three pillows now.
9. Three months ago, I needed only one pillow.
10. Over the past 2 months, I have put on about 10 pounds.
11. My legs are swollen at the end of the day.
12. My appetite is poor.
13. I do not have recent chest pain.
14. I do not have nausea or vomiting.
15. I had a heart attack 5 years ago and was hospitalized for 7 days.
16. I have had high blood pressure for 25 years.
17. I have had high cholesterol for 15 years.
18. I take digoxin 0.25 mg daily, hydrochlorothiazide 50 mg daily, atenolol 50 mg daily, simvastatin 20 mg daily, and aspirin daily.
19. I have no allergies.
20. I have smoked 1½ packs per day for the past 35 years. I can't seem to stop, not even after my heart attack.
21. My father died of a stroke at age 74.

PHYSICAL CHECKLIST

1. Took blood pressure
2. Performed ophthalmoscopic examination
3. Evaluated anterior lung fields by tactile fremitus (4 levels)
4. Evaluated anterior lung fields by percussion (4 levels)
5. Evaluated anterior lung fields by auscultation
6. Evaluated posterior lung fields by tactile fremitus (4 levels)
7. Evaluated posterior lung fields by percussion (4 levels)
8. Evaluated posterior lung fields by auscultation
9. Evaluated heart by auscultation (4 positions)
10. Evaluated liver size by palpation

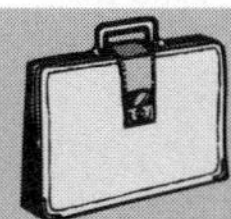

SP's Communication and Interpersonal Skills (CIS) Checklist

1. Knocked before entering
2. Opened interview by introducing self
3. Addressed patient using last name with introduction (e.g., Ms. Balcomb)
4. Appearance (e.g., clean and neat)
5. Allowed patient to express reason for seeking medical attention
6. Made comfortable eye contact
7. Did *not* use leading/biased questions (e.g., "You don't have…" or "You're not…")
8. Asked questions individually
9. Did *not* use the "Why" question
10. Concentrated and focused on patient's needs
11. Maintained comfortable and appropriate distance
12. Gave patient time to think and answer without interrupting
13. Used proper draping during physical exam
14. Did physical examination in an orderly manner
15. Summarized patient's condition (or asked patient to summarize)
16. Discussed diagnostic tests and/or next step in treatment in lay terms
17. Asked whether patient had other questions/concerns
18. Provided patient education/suggestions where appropriate
19. Did *not* give false reassurances
20. Showed empathy

123 SP's Spoken English Proficiency (SEP) Rating Scale

	Poor	Fair	Good	Very Good	Excellent
1. Ability of *patient* to understand *candidate*	1	2	3	4	5
2. Ability of *candidate* to understand *patient*	1	2	3	4	5
3. Candidate is articulate	1	2	3	4	5
4. Words are pronounced correctly	1	2	3	4	5
5. Range of vocabulary and sentence structure	1	2	3	4	5
6. Stress, rhythm, and intonation	1	2	3	4	5
7. Grammar	1	2	3	4	5
8. Repair strategies	1	2	3	4	5

Example of a Satisfactory Patient Note (PN)

HISTORY—Include any significant pertinent positives and negatives

Ms. Betty Balcomb is a 65-year-old with CAD (S/P MI 5 years ago) who presents to the clinic with worsening shortness of breath.

HISTORY OF PRESENT ILLNESS

- Worsening shortness of breath over the past 3 months
- (+) DOE (dyspnea on exertion)—now, 1 block; 3 months ago, 3–4 blocks
- (+) orthopnea—now, 3 pillows; 3 months ago, 1 pillow
- (+) PND (paroxysmal nocturnal dyspnea) in past week
- (+) 10-pound weight gain in past 2 months
- (+) edema at the end of the day
- (+) decreased appetite
- (–) recent chest pain, nausea or vomiting

PAST MEDICAL HISTORY

- (+) MI, 5 years ago; hospitalized for 7 days
- (+) HT × 25 years
- (+) high cholesterol × 15 years
- Medications
  Digoxin 0.25 mg daily
  Hydrochlorothiazide (HCTZ) 50 mg daily
  Atenolol 50 mg daily
  Simvastatin 20 mg daily
  Aspirin daily
- (–) allergies

SOCIAL HISTORY

- Retired librarian
- Married, 2 sons, ages 39 and 41
- Smokes 1½ packs per day for the past 35 years
- Decreased libido "for some time"

FAMILY HISTORY

- Mother died—"old age," age 85
- Father died—stroke, age 74
- Sister died—multiple myeloma, age 63

REVIEW OF SYSTEMS

- Noncontributory

PHYSICAL EXAMINATION—Include any significant pertinent positives and negatives

GENERAL

- Physical examination reveals a well-developed, obese, 65-year-old woman appearing her stated age, complaining of shortness of breath, and in mild-moderate respiratory distress

VITAL SIGNS

- BP 160/85
- Otherwise WNL

HEAD, EARS, EYES, NOSE, AND THROAT

- Optic discs clear with sharp disc margins; color WNL; vasculature WNL

CHEST

- Clear to P&A anteriorly and posteriorly

HEART

- PMI 5th ICS, MCL
- S_1S_2 WNL
- (+) S_3
- (–) murmurs or rubs

ABDOMEN

- (+) BS
- (–) hepatosplenomegaly (liver span 10 cm in MCL)

DIFFERENTIAL DIAGNOSIS

In order of likelihood, write no more than five (5) differential diagnoses

1. Congestive heart failure
2. Diastolic cardiac dysfunction
3. COPD
4. Pneumonia
5. Pulmonary emboli

DIAGNOSTIC WORKUP

Immediate plans, write no more than five (5) diagnostic studies

1. Chest x-ray
2. ECG
3. Echocardiogram
4. CBC, BUN, creatinine
5. V/Q scan pending above studies

CASE 17—Mr. Barry Pinchet

Mr. Barry Pinchet, a 74-year-old man, presents to clinic complaining of confusion.

VITAL SIGNS

Temperature: 98.6° F	**Pulse:** 80 regular
Blood Pressure: 150/85	**Respiratory Rate:** 12 regular

EXAMINEE'S TASKS

In the next 15 minutes, you are to:

1. Take a focused history
2. Do a focused physical examination
3. Discuss your initial clinical impressions and workup plans with the patient
4. Write the Patient Note after leaving the room

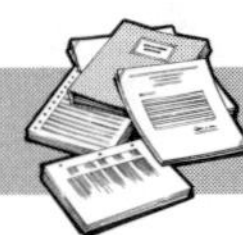

Examinee's Data Gathering (DG) Checklists

HISTORY CHECKLIST

1. ______
2. ______
3. ______
4. ______
5. ______
6. ______
7. ______
8. ______
9. ______
10. ______
11. ______
12. ______
13. ______
14. ______
15. ______
16. ______
17. ______
18. ______
19. ______
20. ______

PHYSICAL EXAMINATION CHECKLIST

1. ______
2. ______
3. ______
4. ______
5. ______
6. ______
7. ______
8. ______

9. ______________________________
10. ______________________________
11. ______________________________

Total DG Score ______ *Passing Score for DG is 22 points (70%)*

Examinee's Communication and Interpersonal Skills (CIS) Checklist

1. ______________________________
2. ______________________________
3. ______________________________
4. ______________________________
5. ______________________________
6. ______________________________
7. ______________________________
8. ______________________________
9. ______________________________
10. ______________________________
11. ______________________________
12. ______________________________
13. ______________________________
14. ______________________________
15. ______________________________
16. ______________________________
17. ______________________________
18. ______________________________
19. ______________________________
20. ______________________________

Total CIS Score ______ *Passing Score for CIS is 14 points (70%)*

123 Examinee's Spoken English Proficiency (SEP) Rating Scale

	Poor	Fair	Good	Very Good	Excellent
1. Ability of *patient* to understand *candidate*	1	2	3	4	5
2. Ability of *candidate* to understand *patient*	1	2	3	4	5
3. Candidate is articulate	1	2	3	4	5
4. Words are pronounced correctly	1	2	3	4	5
5. Range of vocabulary and sentence structure	1	2	3	4	5
6. Stress, rhythm, and intonation	1	2	3	4	5
7. Grammar	1	2	3	4	5
8. Repair strategies	1	2	3	4	5

Total SEP Score ______ *Passing Score for SEP is 28 points (70%)*

Examinee's Patient Note (PN)

HISTORY—Include any significant pertinent positives and negatives

PHYSICAL EXAMINATION—Include any significant pertinent positives and negatives

DIFFERENTIAL DIAGNOSIS

In order of likelihood, write no more than five (5) differential diagnoses

1.
2.
3.
4.
5.

DIAGNOSTIC WORKUP

Immediate plans, write no more than five (5) diagnostic studies

1.
2.
3.
4.
5.

Background Information for Standardized Patient

PATIENT BEHAVIOR

Eyes dart around the room; keeps resettling himself in the chair; smiles a lot

AFFECT

Looks confused; is very pleasant

PROVOCATIVE QUESTION(S) AND PLAUSIBLE ANSWER(S)

"I'm not sure why my son wanted me to come here. Will this take long?"

"I am glad that you have come in today. I'll get you back home real soon."

ADDITIONAL NOTES

The patient answers all questions slowly after thinking about the question; constantly says, in answer to many questions, "Not more than anyone else my age"; his son is outside answering a telephone call but will come in shortly. Patient wears two different shoes and his underwear is on inside out.

CHIEF COMPLAINT

"My son thinks I'm confused."

HISTORY OF PRESENT ILLNESS

Barry Pinchet is a 74-year-old man who was brought in by his son for evaluation of confusion and forgetfulness, but he really feels fine. He shows you a piece of paper with a note written by his son. The note says, "I've noticed that my Dad has been confused at times over the past 1–2 years. He also has fallen several times at home in the past 2–3 months, and I am worried about him. I'll be right in."

He has no history of head trauma; he denies having fallen. He says his son is wrong.

He says that he really is not confused any more than others his age. He says that he has no problem remembering things.

He has no history of dizziness (except when he gets up quickly), weakness, seizures, incontinence, visual problems, or walking problems. He is not sad or depressed. He loves going to the library and reading to the children. His son lives about 20 minutes away and visits him about twice a week.

He says that he has no problem bathing, walking, or dressing. He does remember getting lost on the bus. He took the wrong number and when he got off, he couldn't find how to get home so he called his son who found him and brought him home. He uses only a cell phone now, which his son pays for, because his land line was disconnected (he had forgotten to pay his bill). His son pays his rent now because he forgets to pay that bill as well, but says that's normal for someone his age. His son helps him with the shopping as he has arthritis of his back and can't "carry the…the…the…oh yeah, packages". His son says his house is a mess and things are always moved around.

PAST MEDICAL HISTORY

He doesn't remember any problems except the arthritis of his back.

MEDICATIONS

He has a list that he hands to the doctor (looks very well worn, and is folded into a small rectangle).

ALLERGIES

He doesn't think he has any.

SOCIAL HISTORY

He retired a while ago. He was a house painter. He used to smoke and drink beer, but his son doesn't give him money for this, so he hasn't smoked or drunk beer in a while.

FAMILY HISTORY

His parents died a while ago. He thinks that they were in good health.

SEXUAL HISTORY

He has not been sexually active since his wife died. He doesn't remember how long ago it was.

REVIEW OF SYSTEMS

Noncontributory

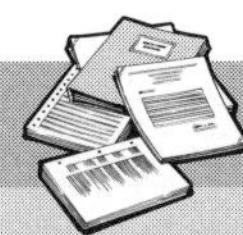

SP's Data Gathering (DG) Checklists

HISTORY CHECKLIST

1. My son brought me here today.
2. My son says that I am confused and forgetful; I really feel fine.
3. Here's a note from my son....
4. I have no history of head injury.
5. I have not fallen.
6. I am not more confused than others my age.
7. I do not have problems remembering things.
8. I do not have any dizziness, except when I get up quickly.
9. I do not have weakness.
10. I do not have seizures.
11. I have never had loss of urine or bowel function.
12. I have no visual problems
13. I have no walking problems.
14. I am not sad or depressed.
15. I love going to the library and reading to the children.
16. My son lives about 20 minutes away and visits me about twice a week.
17. I have no problem bathing, walking, or dressing (*any 2 items*).
18. I did get lost once when I was on a bus.
19. My telephone was disconnected because they said I didn't pay the bill.
20. My son helps me with the shopping as I have arthritis of my back.

PHYSICAL CHECKLIST

1. Evaluated for orthostatic hypotension
2. Evaluated pupils
3. Evaluated EOMs
4. Performed ophthalmoscopic examination
5. Evaluated carotids by auscultation
6. Evaluated thyroid (anteriorly and posteriorly)
7. Evaluated heart by auscultation
8. Evaluated DTRs in lower extremities
9. Evaluated cerebellar function (Romberg, heel-to-shin, or finger-to-nose)
10. Evaluated orientation to person, time, and place
11. Assessed at least 3 items on mini-mental examination

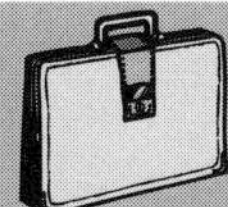

SP's Communication and Interpersonal Skills (CIS) Checklist

1. Knocked before entering
2. Opened interview by introducing self
3. Addressed patient using last name with introduction (e.g., Mr. Pinchet)
4. Appearance (e.g., clean and neat)
5. Allowed patient to express reason for seeking medical attention
6. Made comfortable eye contact
7. Did *not* use leading/biased questions (e.g., "You don't have…" or "You're not…")
8. Asked questions individually
9. Did *not* use the "Why" question
10. Concentrated and focused on patient's needs
11. Maintained comfortable and appropriate distance
12. Gave patient time to think and answer without interrupting
13. Used proper draping during physical exam
14. Did physical examination in an orderly manner
15. Summarized patient's condition (or asked patient to summarize)
16. Discussed diagnostic tests and/or next step in treatment in lay terms
17. Asked whether patient had other questions/concerns
18. Provided patient education/suggestions where appropriate
19. Did *not* give false assurances
20. Showed empathy

123 SP's Spoken English Proficiency (SEP) Rating Scale

	Poor	Fair	Good	Very Good	Excellent
1. Ability of *patient* to understand *candidate*	1	2	3	4	5
2. Ability of *candidate* to understand *patient*	1	2	3	4	5
3. Candidate is articulate	1	2	3	4	5
4. Words are pronounced correctly	1	2	3	4	5
5. Range of vocabulary and sentence structure	1	2	3	4	5
6. Stress, rhythm, and intonation	1	2	3	4	5
7. Grammar	1	2	3	4	5
8. Repair strategies	1	2	3	4	5

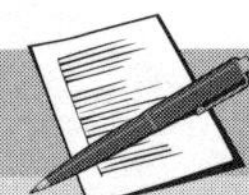

Example of a Satisfactory Patient Note (PN)

HISTORY—Include any significant pertinent positives and negatives

Mr. Barry Pinchet is a 74-year-old man brought in by his son for evaluation of confusion and forgetfulness. The patient presented me with a note from the son stating, "I've noticed that my Dad has been become confused at times over the past 1–2 years. He also has fallen several times at home in the past 2–3 months, and I am worried about him."

HISTORY OF PRESENT ILLNESS

- Denies having fallen or being confused. Says he doesn't think he is more confused than anyone else his age
- (–) history of head trauma
- (–) problem remembering things
- (–) dizziness, except when the patient gets up quickly
- (–) weakness, seizures, incontinence of urinary or bowel function
- (–) visual problems
- (–) walking problems
- (–) depression; loves going to the library and reading to the children

PAST MEDICAL HISTORY

- (+) arthritis of back
- Medications
  Atenolol 50 mg daily
  Cimetidine 200 mg q6h for heartburn
  Atorvastatin 40 mg daily
  Aspirin
- (–) allergies

SOCIAL HISTORY

- Retired house painter
- Wife died a while ago; one son, age?
- Son lives about 20 minutes away and visits him about twice a week
- No problem with bathing, walking, or dressing
- Telephone was disconnected because he didn't pay the bill
- Son helps with shopping

FAMILY HISTORY

- Parents deceased—? cause

REVIEW OF SYSTEMS

- Noncontributory

PHYSICAL EXAMINATION—Include any significant pertinent positives and negatives

GENERAL

- Physical examination reveals a well-developed, slightly obese, 74-year-old man, appearing older than his stated age, who was brought in by his son, stating that his father is confused and forgetful

VITAL SIGNS

- BP 150/85
- (–) orthostatic changes
- Otherwise WNL

HEAD, EARS, EYES, NOSE, AND THROAT

- PERRL
- EOMs intact
- Right eye (OD)—disc clear with sharp disc margins; color WNL; vasculature WNL
- Left eye (OS)—poorly visualized due to central lenticular opacity
- Carotids—no bruits present
- Thyroid—no masses felt or bruit heard

HEART

- PMI 6th ICS-MCL
- S_1S_2 WNL
- (–) murmurs, gallops, or rubs heard

NEUROLOGICAL

- Oriented × 3
- Mini-Mental—unable to recall 3 objects correctly; unable to follow 3-step command
- DTRs 2+ bilaterally—upper and lower extremities
- Gait—patient refused due to extreme dizziness
- (–) Romberg

DIFFERENTIAL DIAGNOSIS

In order of likelihood, write no more than five (5) differential diagnoses

1. Alzheimer's disease
2. Multi-infarct dementia
3. Subdural hematoma
4. Intracranial tumor
5. Hypothyroidism

DIAGNOSTIC WORKUP

Immediate plans, write no more than five (5) diagnostic studies

1. CT of head
2. MRI of brain
3. CBC, glucose, TSH, serum B_{12}, BUN, creatinine, Ca^{2+}, AST, ALT, alkaline phosphatase, bilirubin, VDRL, RPR
4. EEG
5. ______________________________

CASE 18—Mr. Vinny Maoli

Mr. Vinny Maoli, a 36-year-old man, presents to clinic complaining of worsening cough.

VITAL SIGNS

Temperature: 101.2° F	**Pulse:** 90 regular
Blood Pressure: 155/85	**Respiratory Rate:** 18 regular

EXAMINEE'S TASKS

In the next 15 minutes, you are to:

1) Take a focused history
2) Do a focused physical examination
3) Discuss your initial clinical impressions and workup plans with the patient
4) Write the Patient Note after leaving the room

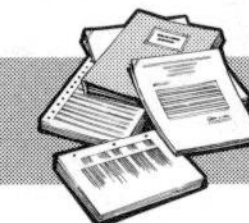

Examinee's Data Gathering (DG) Checklists

HISTORY CHECKLIST

1. ______
2. ______
3. ______
4. ______
5. ______
6. ______
7. ______
8. ______
9. ______
10. ______
11. ______
12. ______
13. ______
14. ______
15. ______
16. ______
17. ______
18. ______
19. ______
20. ______
21. ______
22. ______
23. ______
24. ______

PHYSICAL EXAMINATION CHECKLIST

1. ______
2. ______
3. ______

4. ______
5. ______
6. ______
7. ______
8. ______
9. ______
10. ______

Total DG Score ______ *Passing Score for DG is 24 points (70%)*

Examinee's Communication and Interpersonal Skills (CIS) Checklist

1. ______
2. ______
3. ______
4. ______
5. ______
6. ______
7. ______
8. ______
9. ______
10. ______
11. ______
12. ______
13. ______
14. ______
15. ______
16. ______

17. ______________________________
18. ______________________________
19. ______________________________
20. ______________________________

Total CIS Score ______ *Passing Score for CIS is 14 points (70%)*

123 Examinee's Spoken English Proficiency (SEP) Rating Scale

	Poor	Fair	Good	Very Good	Excellent
1. Ability of *patient* to understand *candidate*	1	2	3	4	5
2. Ability of *candidate* to understand *patient*	1	2	3	4	5
3. Candidate is articulate	1	2	3	4	5
4. Words are pronounced correctly	1	2	3	4	5
5. Range of vocabulary and sentence structure	1	2	3	4	5
6. Stress, rhythm, and intonation	1	2	3	4	5
7. Grammar	1	2	3	4	5
8. Repair strategies	1	2	3	4	5

Total SEP Score ______ *Passing Score for SEP is 28 points (70%)*

Examinee's Patient Note (PN)

HISTORY—Include any significant pertinent positives and negatives

PHYSICAL EXAMINATION— Include any significant pertinent positives and negatives

DIFFERENTIAL DIAGNOSIS

In order of likelihood, write no more than five (5) differential diagnoses

1.
2.
3.
4.
5.

DIAGNOSTIC WORKUP

Immediate plans, write no more than five (5) diagnostic studies

1.
2.
3.
4.
5.

Background Information for Standardized Patient

PATIENT BEHAVIOR

Tapping feet; tapping fingers; perhaps biting fingernails; cough every 3–4 minutes during the encounter

AFFECT

Nervous; on edge

PROVOCATIVE QUESTION(S) AND PLAUSIBLE ANSWER(S)

"What the hell is wrong with me? I mean, a cough is one thing, but now I've got blood.... I'm getting real worried!"

"Let me first ask you some questions and do a few tests to determine what's going on. I promise you that I will give you something as soon as I have a better idea of your medical problem."

Remember that what appears on the presenting situation is only the tip of the iceberg, and you cannot tell what is really going on with a patient until you ask them good open-ended questions.

CHIEF COMPLAINT

"This cough is getting worse and worse."

HISTORY OF PRESENT ILLNESS

Vinny Maoli is a 36-year-old man who comes to clinic for evaluation of worsening cough for the past 1–2 months. He first noticed it about 2½ months ago after having spent about 3 years on a farm in rural Georgia where he worked for a bulldozing company. He thought that it was "like a flu thing." The cough started as a dry hacking cough. His cough is nonproductive, but just recently he noted some blood-streaked sputum. He has never coughed up clots of blood. He has noted that his exercise tolerance has decreased; he now gets short of breath after walking about 2 blocks. Two months ago, he had no trouble walking at all. He has had a low-grade fever to 101° F on and off for the past month. He also has had a 22-pound weight loss in the past 2 months; he was not trying to lose weight, but his appetite is down. On occasion, he has had dull headaches over the front of his head, which have improved with Tylenol. He has right-sided chest pain when he takes a big breath.

PAST MEDICAL HISTORY

Appendectomy, age 14

MEDICATIONS

None

ALLERGIES

None

SOCIAL HISTORY

He is a 2-pack-per-day smoker for the past 16 years. He has been a farm worker since he was 17 years old. He enjoys having 2–3 six packs of beer per week with the guys.

FAMILY HISTORY

His parents are both alive; his mother is 55 years old and has high blood pressure; his father is 56 years old and has diabetes. He has one older brother, age 38, who is in good health.

SEXUAL HISTORY

He is gay and has had many partners over the years. He now has three partners and has anal and oral intercourse with them. He uses condoms when he remembers. He was tested for HIV 4 years ago; it was negative. He has had the "clap" (gonorrhea) twice (ages 21 and 29) and was treated with penicillin. Two of his partners died of AIDS; he learned about one of them just 3 months ago.

REVIEW OF SYSTEMS

He has frequent sore throats.

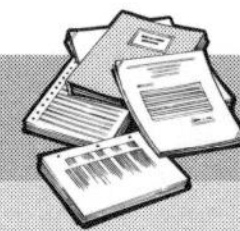

SP's Data Gathering (DG) Checklists

HISTORY CHECKLIST

1. This cough is getting worse and worse.
2. I first noticed the cough about 2½ months ago.
3. I spent about 3 years on a farm in rural Georgia where I worked for a bulldozing company.
4. It started like a flulike syndrome.
5. The cough is nonproductive of sputum.
6. Just recently, I noted some blood-streaked sputum.
7. My exercise tolerance has decreased; I now get short of breath after walking about 2 blocks.
8. Two months ago, I had no trouble walking at all.
9. I have had a low-grade fever to 101° F on and off for the past month.
10. I've lost 22 pounds in the past 2 months.
11. I just don't seem to have any appetite.
12. On occasion, I have had dull headaches over the front of my head, which have improved with Tylenol.
13. I have right-sided chest pain when I take a big breath.
14. I am a 2-pack-per-day smoker for the past 16 years.
15. I have been a farm worker since I was 17 years old.
16. I am gay and have had many partners over the years.
17. I have anal and oral intercourse.
18. I use condoms when I remember.
19. I was tested for HIV 4 years ago; it was negative.
20. I had the "clap" twice and was treated with penicillin.
21. Two of my partners died of AIDS.
22. I have frequent sore throats.
23. I am not taking any medications.
24. I have no allergies.

PHYSICAL CHECKLIST

1. Evaluated for head and neck lymphadenopathy by palpation
2. Performed ophthalmoscopic examination
3. Inspected posterior pharynx.
4. Evaluated anterior chest by percussion (4 levels)

5. Evaluated anterior chest by auscultation (4 levels)
6. Evaluated posterior chest by percussion (4 levels)
7. Evaluated posterior chest by auscultation (4 levels)
8. Evaluated heart by auscultation (4 levels)
9. Evaluated liver size
10. Evaluated spleen for organomegaly

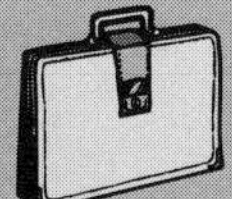

SP's Communication and Interpersonal Skills (CIS) Checklist

1. Knocked before entering
2. Opened interview by introducing self
3. Addressed patient using last name with introduction (e.g., Mr. Maoli)
4. Appearance (e.g., clean and neat)
5. Allowed patient to express reason for seeking medical attention
6. Made comfortable eye contact
7. Did *not* use leading/biased questions (e.g., "You don't have…" or "You're not…")
8. Asked questions individually
9. Did *not* use the "Why" question
10. Concentrated and focused on patient's needs
11. Maintained comfortable and appropriate distance
12. Gave patient time to think and answer without interrupting
13. Used proper draping during physical exam
14. Did physical examination in an orderly manner
15. Summarized patient's condition (or asked patient to summarize)
16. Discussed diagnostic tests and/or next step in treatment in lay terms
17. Asked whether patient had other questions/concerns
18. Provided patient education/suggestions where appropriate
19. Did *not* give false assurances
20. Showed empathy

123 SP's Spoken English Proficiency (SEP) Rating Scale

	Poor	Fair	Good	Very Good	Excellent
1. Ability of *patient* to understand *candidate*	1	2	3	4	5
2. Ability of *candidate* to understand *patient*	1	2	3	4	5
3. Candidate is articulate	1	2	3	4	5
4. Words are pronounced correctly	1	2	3	4	5
5. Range of vocabulary and sentence structure	1	2	3	4	5
6. Stress, rhythm, and intonation	1	2	3	4	5
7. Grammar	1	2	3	4	5
8. Repair strategies	1	2	3	4	5

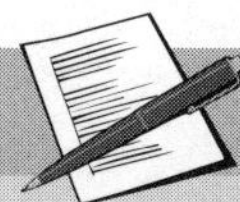

Example of a Satisfactory Patient Note (PN)

HISTORY—Include any significant pertinent positives and negatives

Mr. Vinny Maoli is a 36-year-old gay man who presents to clinic with the chief complaint of "this cough is getting worse and worse."

HISTORY OF PRESENT ILLNESS

- Cough started about 2½ months ago as a flulike illness
- Cough is nonproductive of sputum; just recently, some blood-streaked sputum
- Short of breath now after walking about 2 blocks; 2 months ago, no trouble walking
- (+) low-grade fever to 101° F for past month
- (+) 22-pound weight loss in past 2 months; no appetite
- On occasion, dull headaches over the front of his head, which have improved with Tylenol
- (+) right-sided chest pain with big breath

PAST MEDICAL HISTORY

- (+) H/O gonorrhea × 2 ages 21 and 29; treated with penicillin
- (+) appendectomy, age 14
- (−) medications
- (−) allergies

SOCIAL HISTORY

- Gay man with many partners over the years
- Has anal and oral intercourse
- Uses condoms "when he remembers"
- Tested for HIV 4 years ago; it was negative
- Two partners died of AIDS
- Recently returned from 3 years working on a farm in rural Georgia for a bulldozing company
- Farm worker since age 17
- (+) 2 ppd cigarette smoker for 16 years

FAMILY HISTORY

- Mother—55 years old, high blood pressure
- Father—56 years old, diabetes
- Brother—38 years old, A&W

REVIEW OF SYSTEMS

- (+) frequent sore throats

PHYSICAL EXAMINATION—Include any significant pertinent positives and negatives

GENERAL

- Physical examination reveals a well-developed, thin, 36-year-old man appearing older than his stated age and coughing

VITAL SIGNS

- BP 155/85
- 101.2° F
- Respirations 18/minute
- HR 90 regular

HEAD, EARS, EYES, NOSE, AND THROAT

- (+) posterior cervical, tonsillar, and superficial cervical adenopathy; several 1-cm nodes slightly tender, not matted, not fixed to overlying or underlying tissue
- Optic discs clear with sharp disc margins; color WNL; vasculature WNL; (–) hemorrhages, exudates
- Posterior pharynx without erythema or exudates

CHEST

- Clear to P&A

HEART

- PMI 5th ICS-MCL
- S_1S_2 WNL
- (–) murmurs, gallops, or rubs

ABDOMEN

- (–) hepatosplenomegaly

DIFFERENTIAL DIAGNOSIS

In order of likelihood, write no more than five (5) differential diagnoses

1. AIDS
2. *Pneumocystis carinii* pneumonia
3. Histoplasmosis
4. Tuberculosis
5. Cryptococcosis

DIAGNOSTIC WORKUP

Immediate plans, write no more than five (5) diagnostic studies

1. Chest x-ray
2. CBC, HIV antibody, arterial blood gas, CO_2, LDH, alkaline phosphatase, ALT, complement-fixing antibodies for histoplasmosis, CD4 lymphocyte count
3. Sputum for culture, Gram stain, PCP analysis, and acid-fast bacillus smear × 3
4. PPD
5. Bronchoscopy with bronchoalveolar lavage and biopsy

CASE 19—Ms. Mei Ling

Ms. Mei Ling, a 41-year-old woman, presents to clinic complaining of rectal bleeding.

VITAL SIGNS

Temperature: 98.6° F	**Pulse:** 70 regular
Blood Pressure: 115/65	**Respiratory Rate:** 12 regular

EXAMINEE'S TASKS

In the next 15 minutes, you are to:

1. Take a focused history
2. Do a focused physical examination
3. Discuss your initial clinical impressions and workup plans with the patient
4. Write the Patient Note after leaving the room

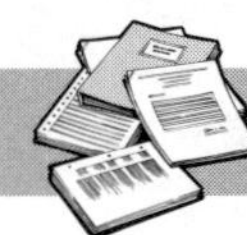

Examinee's Data Gathering (DG) Checklists

HISTORY CHECKLIST

1. ______
2. ______
3. ______
4. ______
5. ______
6. ______
7. ______
8. ______
9. ______
10. ______
11. ______
12. ______
13. ______
14. ______
15. ______
16. ______
17. ______
18. ______
19. ______
20. ______

PHYSICAL EXAMINATION CHECKLIST

1. ______
2. ______
3. ______
4. ______
5. ______
6. ______

7. ____
8. ____

Total DG Score _____ *Passing Score for DG is 20 points (70%)*

Examinee's Communication and Interpersonal Skills (CIS) Checklist

1. ____
2. ____
3. ____
4. ____
5. ____
6. ____
7. ____
8. ____
9. ____
10. ____
11. ____
12. ____
13. ____
14. ____
15. ____
16. ____
17. ____
18. ____
19. ____
20. ____

Total CIS Score _____ *Passing Score for CIS is 14 points (70%)*

123 Examinee's Spoken English Proficiency (SEP) Rating Scale

	Poor	Fair	Good	Very Good	Excellent
1. Ability of *patient* to understand *candidate*	1	2	3	4	5
2. Ability of *candidate* to understand *patient*	1	2	3	4	5
3. Candidate is articulate	1	2	3	4	5
4. Words are pronounced correctly	1	2	3	4	5
5. Range of vocabulary and sentence structure	1	2	3	4	5
6. Stress, rhythm, and intonation	1	2	3	4	5
7. Grammar	1	2	3	4	5
8. Repair strategies	1	2	3	4	5

Total SEP Score ______ *Passing Score for SEP is 28 points (70%)*

Background Information for Standardized Patient

PATIENT BEHAVIOR
Nervous; biting nails; picking at her fingers

AFFECT
Worried

PROVOCATIVE QUESTION(S) AND PLAUSIBLE ANSWER(S)
"Do I have cancer like my mother?

It's too early to say. Let's get some tests first, and then we'll have a better idea."

CHIEF COMPLAINT
"I've got blood in my stool. I'm so scared!"

HISTORY OF PRESENT ILLNESS
Mei Ling is a 41-year-old Asian American woman who comes to clinic with the complaint of blood in her stool. For the past 2 weeks, she has noted blood in her stools every time she has a bowel movement. The blood is mixed in with the stools and on the toilet paper. She also has had diarrhea for the past 2 weeks and has a feeling that she has to move her bowels all the time. Although she has not tried to lose weight, she has lost about 5 pounds in the past month. She has no mucus in the stool. She has no fever, chills, abdominal pain, sick contacts, or recent travel. She was always prone to constipation and used to take Dulcolax before the diarrhea began.

She had a urinary tract infection about a month ago, and her gynecologist gave her an antibiotic for 7 days. She doesn't remember its name.

The timing of a patient's visit to a doctor can be most informative. Why did the patient wait 2 weeks before coming to see a doctor for what might very well be a serious condition, i.e., blood in the stool? The answer is fear. Most patients have something they are fearful of. Assuring them, appropriately, goes a long way toward healing them.

PAST MEDICAL HISTORY
She had a pregnancy termination about 8 years ago.

MEDICATIONS
Multivitamins
Aspirin

ALLERGIES
None

SOCIAL HISTORY
She has never smoked. She doesn't use alcohol or other recreational drugs.

FAMILY HISTORY

Her mother had colon cancer at age 59 and had a colostomy. She now has a "pouch." Her mother is now 65 and doing well. Her father, age 69, has high blood pressure and a lot of allergies.

SEXUAL HISTORY

She is single and is not currently sexually active. She is now a lesbian.

REVIEW OF SYSTEMS

Noncontributory

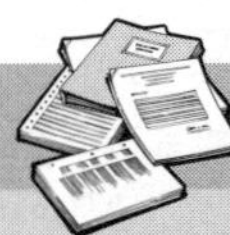

SP's Data Gathering (DG) Checklists

HISTORY CHECKLIST

1. I've got blood in my stool.
2. I've noted blood in my stools for the past 2 weeks.
3. There's been blood in my stools every time I have a bowel movement.
4. The blood is mixed in with the stools and on the toilet paper.
5. I've had diarrhea for the past 2 weeks.
6. I have a feeling that I have to move my bowels all the time.
7. I've lost about 5 pounds in the past month.
8. I have not been trying to lose weight.
9. I have not noticed any mucus in the stool.
10. I have not had any fever or chills.
11. I have not had abdominal pain.
12. I do not have any sick contacts.
13. I have not traveled recently.
14. I have always been prone to constipation.
15. I used to take Dulcolax for the constipation.
16. I had a urinary tract infection about a month ago.
17. My gynecologist gave me an antibiotic to take for 7 days.
18. I am not on any medications other than multivitamins and aspirin.
19. I have no allergies.
20. My mother had colon cancer.

PHYSICAL CHECKLIST

1. Took blood pressure
2. Evaluated for orthostatic hypotension
3. Evaluated heart by auscultation
4. Evaluated bowel sounds by auscultation
5. Performed light palpation of the abdomen in all 4 quadrants *after* auscultation
6. Performed deep palpation of the abdomen in all 4 quadrants
7. Percussed abdomen in all 4 quadrants
8. Evaluated liver for hepatomegaly

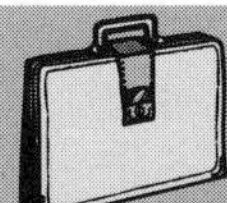

SP's Communication and Interpersonal Skills (CIS) Checklist

1. Knocked before entering
2. Opened interview by introducing self
3. Addressed patient using last name with introduction (e.g., Ms. Ling)
4. Appearance (e.g., clean and neat)
5. Allowed patient to express reason for seeking medical attention
6. Made comfortable eye contact
7. Did *not* use leading/biased questions (e.g., "You don't have..." or "You're not...")
8. Asked questions individually
9. Did *not* use the "Why" question
10. Concentrated and focused on patient's needs
11. Maintained comfortable and appropriate distance
12. Gave patient time to think and answer without interrupting
13. Used proper draping during physical exam
14. Did physical examination in an orderly manner
15. Summarized patient's condition (or asked patient to summarize)
16. Discussed diagnostic tests and/or next step in treatment in lay terms
17. Asked whether patient had other questions/concerns
18. Provided patient education/suggestions where appropriate
19. Did *not* give false assurances
20. Showed empathy

123 SP's Spoken English Proficiency (SEP) Rating Scale

	Poor	Fair	Good	Very Good	Excellent
1. Ability of *patient* to understand *candidate*	1	2	3	4	5
2. Ability of *candidate* to understand *patient*	1	2	3	4	5
3. Candidate is articulate	1	2	3	4	5
4. Words are pronounced correctly	1	2	3	4	5
5. Range of vocabulary and sentence structure	1	2	3	4	5
6. Stress, rhythm, and intonation	1	2	3	4	5
7. Grammar	1	2	3	4	5
8. Repair strategies	1	2	3	4	5

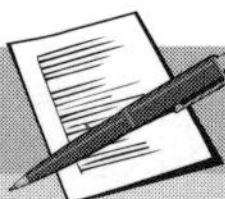

Example of a Satisfactory Patient Note (PN)

HISTORY—Include any significant pertinent positives and negatives

Ms. Mei Ling is a 41-year-old woman with a family history of colon cancer who presents with the chief complaint of "blood in her stool. I'm so scared."

HISTORY OF PRESENT ILLNESS

- (+) blood in stools for past 2 weeks
- Blood in stools with every bowel movement
- Blood mixed with stools and on toilet paper
- (+) diarrhea for the past 2 weeks
- (+) tenesmus
- 5-pound weight loss in past month; not trying to lose weight
- (−) mucus, fever, chills, abdominal pain, no sick contacts, recent travel
- (+) prone previously to constipation and used Dulcolax
- (+) urinary tract infection about a month ago and given antibiotic (name ?) for 7 days
- (−) medications other than multivitamins and aspirin

PAST MEDICAL HISTORY

- Pregnancy termination, 8 years ago
- (−) allergies

SOCIAL HISTORY

- Unmarried, no current relationship
- (−) smoking
- (−) recreational drugs

FAMILY HISTORY

- (+) mother, age 65, had colon cancer at age 59
- Father, age 69, hypertension and allergies

PHYSICAL EXAMINATION—Include any significant pertinent positives and negatives

GENERAL

- Physical examination reveals a thin, 41-year-old woman appearing her stated age and complaining of bloody diarrhea

VITAL SIGNS

- BP 120/70; no orthostatic changes
- Otherwise WNL

HEART

- PMI 5th ICS-MCL
- S_1S_2 WNL
- (–) murmurs, gallops, or rubs

ABDOMEN

- (+) bowel sounds
- (–) tenderness
- (–) masses
- Liver span 10 cm, MCL
- (–) spleen

DIFFERENTIAL DIAGNOSIS

In order of likelihood, write no more than five (5) differential diagnoses

1. Colorectal cancer
2. Diverticulosis
3. Hemorrhoids
4. Pseudomembranous colitis (*Clostridium difficile*)
5. Inflammatory bowel disease

DIAGNOSTIC WORKUP

Immediate plans, write no more than five (5) diagnostic studies

1. Rectal exam and stool for FOBT
2. CBC
3. Stool for *Clostridium difficile* toxin
4. Colonoscopy
5. Stool culture

CASE 20—Ms. Esther Davis

Ms. Esther Davis, a 69-year-old woman, presents to clinic complaining of difficulty in walking.

VITAL SIGNS

Temperature: 98.6° F	**Pulse:** 85 regular
Blood Pressure: 160/85	**Respiratory Rate:** 14 regular

EXAMINEE'S TASKS

In the next 15 minutes, you are to:

1. Take a focused history
2. Do a focused physical examination
3. Discuss your initial clinical impressions and workup plans with the patient
4. Write the Patient Note after leaving the room

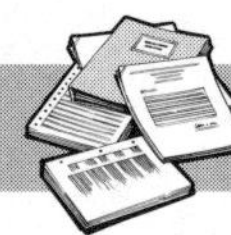

Examinee's Data Gathering (DG) Checklists

HISTORY CHECKLIST

1. ______
2. ______
3. ______
4. ______
5. ______
6. ______
7. ______
8. ______
9. ______
10. ______
11. ______
12. ______
13. ______
14. ______
15. ______
16. ______
17. ______
18. ______
19. ______
20. ______
21. ______
22. ______
23. ______

PHYSICAL EXAMINATION CHECKLIST

1. ______
2. ______
3. ______
4. ______
5. ______

6. ______________________________

7. ______________________________

8. ______________________________

9. ______________________________

10. ______________________________

11. ______________________________

Total DG Score _____ *Passing Score for DG is 24 points (70%)*

Examinee's Communication and Interpersonal Skills (CIS) Checklist

1. ______________________________

2. ______________________________

3. ______________________________

4. ______________________________

5. ______________________________

6. ______________________________

7. ______________________________

8. ______________________________

9. ______________________________

10. ______________________________

11. ______________________________

12. ______________________________

13. ______________________________

14. ______________________________

15. ______________________________

16. ______________________________

17. ______________________________

18. ______________________________

19. ______________________________

20. ______________________________

Total CIS Score _____ *Passing Score for CIS is 14 points (70%)*

123 Examinee's Spoken English Proficiency (SEP) Rating Scale

	Poor	Fair	Good	Very Good	Excellent
1. Ability of *patient* to understand *candidate*	1	2	3	4	5
2. Ability of *candidate* to understand *patient*	1	2	3	4	5
3. Candidate is articulate	1	2	3	4	5
4. Words are pronounced correctly	1	2	3	4	5
5. Range of vocabulary and sentence structure	1	2	3	4	5
6. Stress, rhythm, and intonation	1	2	3	4	5
7. Grammar	1	2	3	4	5
8. Repair strategies	1	2	3	4	5

Total SEP Score ______ *Passing Score for SEP is 28 points (70%)*

Examinee's Patient Note (PN)

HISTORY—Include any significant pertinent positives and negatives

PHYSICAL EXAMINATION—Include any significant pertinent positives and negatives

DIFFERENTIAL DIAGNOSIS

In order of likelihood, write no more than five (5) differential diagnoses

1.
2.
3.
4.
5.

DIAGNOSTIC WORKUP

Immediate plans, write no more than five (5) diagnostic studies

1.
2.
3.
4.
5.

Background Information for Standardized Patient

PATIENT BEHAVIOR

Shuffling gait; hand tremor (which she claims is "…very embarrassing," but "all old people have it")

AFFECT

Sheepish; pleasant

PROVOCATIVE QUESTION(S) AND PLAUSIBLE ANSWER(S)

"This wouldn't mean I have a brain tumor, or anything, Doc, would it?"

"It is good you came in to see me. We will do all the necessary tests to figure out what is going on. It is too soon to tell what is happening, but we will do our very best to help you."

ADDITIONAL NOTES

Shuffling gait; she says that the tremor is very embarrassing, but "all old people have it."

CHIEF COMPLAINT

"I'm having trouble walking and I fell."

HISTORY OF PRESENT ILLNESS

Esther Davis is a 69-year-old woman who comes to clinic today because she is having trouble walking for the past 5–6 months and has fallen several times in the past few weeks. This morning, while preparing breakfast, she tripped and fell in her kitchen. She doesn't think that she hit her head or lost consciousness. She felt a little nauseated but did not vomit. She did not have urinary or bowel incontinence. She was not confused after the event. She did not have chest pain, shortness of breath, or palpitations.

Over the past 5 months, she has noted the development of a tremor of both her hands. She says it is very embarrassing, but "all old people have it." She noticed that it seems to occur when she is not doing anything. When she reaches to do something with her hands, the tremor is less and can even disappear. She drinks only one cup of coffee for breakfast. She doesn't have any other caffeine intake. She does not have numbness of her extremities. She has no history of hot/cold intolerance or palpitations.

She is able to perform her activities of daily living (i.e., feeding, bathing, toileting, dressing) without too much of a problem. She does have some trouble with the instrumental activities of daily living, especially managing her checkbook, shopping, and cooking. Her friend Martha, a neighbor, helps her a lot with her finances and shopping.

PAST MEDICAL HISTORY

She has had chronic obstructive lung disease for about 15 years. She also has a 20-year history of high blood pressure, which is pretty well controlled with medications.

MEDICATIONS

Albuterol inhaler
Theophylline
Atenolol 50 mg daily

ALLERGIES

None

SOCIAL HISTORY

She is a retired employee of the telephone company. She is a widow. Her husband died 2 years ago of a heart attack. She has two sons, ages 45 and 43. Both are well, but they live far away. She smoked more than 2 packs of cigarettes a day for 30 years but stopped after her husband died. She doesn't drink alcohol or use other recreational drugs.

FAMILY HISTORY

Her parents are both dead. She thinks they died of "old age."

SEXUAL HISTORY

She has not been sexually active since her husband's death.

REVIEW OF SYSTEMS

Noncontributory

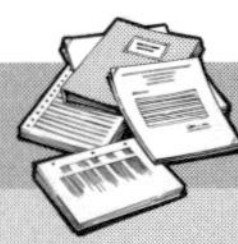

SP's Data Gathering (DG) Checklists

HISTORY CHECKLIST

1. I'm having trouble walking for the past 5 to 6 months.
2. I have fallen several times in the past few weeks.
3. This morning while preparing breakfast, I tripped and fell in my kitchen.
4. I don't think I hit my head.
5. I did not lose consciousness.
6. I felt a little nauseated, but I did not vomit.
7. I did not have urinary or bowel incontinence.
8. I was not confused after the fall.
9. I did not have chest pain.
10. I did not have shortness of breath.
11. I did not have palpitations.
12. Over the past 5 months, I have noted the development of a tremor of both my hands.
13. I have noticed that the tremor seems to occur when I am not doing anything.
14. When I reach to do something with my hands, the tremor is less and can even disappear.
15. I drink only one cup of coffee for breakfast; I do not have any other caffeine intake.
16. I do not have numbness of my extremities.
17. I do not have hot/cold intolerance.
18. I have never had palpitations.
19. I have no problem with eating, bathing, toileting, or dressing myself.
20. I do have a little trouble managing my checkbook, shopping, and cooking.
21. I don't drink alcohol or use recreational drugs.
22. I use an albuterol inhaler, and I take theophylline and atenolol 50 mg daily.
23. I smoked 2 packs of cigarettes a day for 30 years but stopped after my husband died.

PHYSICAL CHECKLIST

1. Took blood pressure
2. Evaluated for orthostatic hypotension
3. Evaluated pupils
4. Evaluated EOMs
5. Evaluated visual fields by confrontation field testing

6. Evaluated the heart by auscultation
7. Evaluated motor strength in lower extremities
8. Evaluated cerebellar function with rapid alternating movement
9. Evaluated DTRs in lower extremities
10. Evaluated gait
11. Evaluated orientation to person, place, and time

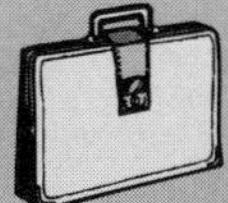

SP's Communication and Interpersonal Skills (CIS) Checklist

1. Knocked before entering
2. Opened interview by introducing self
3. Addressed patient using last name with introduction (e.g., Ms. Davis)
4. Appearance (e.g., clean and neat)
5. Allowed patient to express reason for seeking medical attention
6. Made comfortable eye contact
7. Did *not* use leading/biased questions (e.g., "You don't have…" or "You're not…")
8. Asked questions individually
9. Did *not* use the "Why" question
10. Concentrated and focused on patient's needs
11. Maintained comfortable and appropriate distance
12. Gave patient time to think and answer without interrupting
13. Used proper draping during physical exam
14. Did physical examination in an orderly manner
15. Summarized patient's condition (or asked patient to summarize)
16. Discussed diagnostic tests and/or next step in treatment in lay terms
17. Asked whether patient had other questions/concerns
18. Provided patient education/suggestions where appropriate
19. Did *not* give false assurances
20. Showed empathy

123 SP's Spoken English Proficiency (SEP) Rating Scale

	Poor	Fair	Good	Very Good	Excellent
1. Ability of *patient* to understand *candidate*	1	2	3	4	5
2. Ability of *candidate* to understand *patient*	1	2	3	4	5
3. Candidate is articulate	1	2	3	4	5
4. Words are pronounced correctly	1	2	3	4	5
5. Range of vocabulary and sentence structure	1	2	3	4	5
6. Stress, rhythm, and intonation	1	2	3	4	5
7. Grammar	1	2	3	4	5
8. Repair strategies	1	2	3	4	5

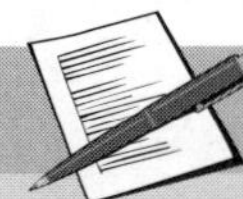

Example of a Satisfactory Patient Note (PN)

HISTORY—Include any significant pertinent positives and negatives

Ms. Esther Davis is a 69-year-old woman who presents to the clinic with the chief complaint of difficulty in walking.

HISTORY OF PRESENT ILLNESS

- Difficulty in walking for the past 5–6 months
- Fell several times in the past few weeks
- "Tripped" and fell in kitchen today while preparing breakfast
- (+) nausea; (–) vomiting
- (–) head injury
- (–) loss of consciousness
- (–) urinary or bowel incontinence
- (–) confusion after the fall
- (–) chest pain, shortness of breath, palpitations
- (–) tremor of hands noticed in the past 5 months, which occurs when patient is not doing anything; when she reaches to do something, the tremor lessens and may disappear
- Caffeine intake—one cup of coffee for breakfast; no other caffeine intake
- (–) numbness of my extremities
- (–) hot/cold intolerance or palpitations

PAST MEDICAL HISTORY

- (+) COPD (chronic obstructive pulmonary disease) × 15 years
- (+) HT × 20 years
- Medications
  Albuterol inhaler as needed
  Theophylline as needed
  Atenolol 50 mg daily
- (–) allergies

SOCIAL HISTORY

- Retired employee of telephone company
- Widow, husband died 2 year ago, MI
- Two sons, ages 45 and 43
- (–) problems with eating, bathing, toileting, or dressing
- Does have a little trouble managing her checkbook, shopping, and cooking
- (–) alcohol or other recreational drug use
- Smoking—60 pack/year history (2 ppd × 30 years) but stopped after husband died

FAMILY HISTORY

- Parents deceased—"old age"

REVIEW OF SYSTEMS

- Noncontributory

PHYSICAL EXAMINATION—Include any significant pertinent positives and negatives

GENERAL

- Physical examination reveals a well-developed, slightly obese, 69-year-old woman appearing her stated age and complaining of difficulty in walking.

VITAL SIGNS

- BP 160/85
- (–) orthostatic changes
- Otherwise WNL

HEAD, EARS, EYES, NOSE, AND THROAT

- PERRL
- EOMs intact
- Visual fields intact
- Optic discs clear with sharp disc margins; color WNL; vasculature WNL

CHEST

- Clear to P&A

CARDIAC

- PMI 5th ICS-MCL
- S_1S_2 WNL
- (–) murmurs, gallops, or rubs

NEUROLOGICAL

- Oriented × 3 to person, place, and time
- Motor strength intact
- DTRs intact (biceps, triceps, patellar, Achilles—all 2+ bilaterally
- (–) Romberg
- Heel-to-toe WNL
- Gait—shuffling

DIFFERENTIAL DIAGNOSIS

In order of likelihood, write no more than five (5) differential diagnoses

1. Parkinson's disease
2. Thyroid disease
3. Familial benign tremor
4. Cardiac syncope
5. Drug-induced tremor

DIAGNOSTIC WORKUP

Immediate plans, write no more than five (5) diagnostic studies

1. CBC, TSH, free T4, glucose, heavy metal screen
2. MRI of brain
3. ECG
4. Holter monitor
5. Echocardiogram

CASE 21—Ms. Susan Bell

Ms. Susan Bell, a 31-year-old woman, presents to clinic complaining of loss of menstrual periods.

VITAL SIGNS

Temperature: 98.6° F	**Pulse:** 80 regular
Blood Pressure: 130/70	**Respiratory Rate:** 12 regular

EXAMINEE'S TASKS

In the next 15 minutes, you are to:

1) Take a focused history
2) Do a focused physical examination
3) Discuss your initial clinical impressions and workup plans with the patient
4) Write the Patient Note after leaving the room

Examinee's Data Gathering (DG) Checklists

HISTORY CHECKLIST

1. _____
2. _____
3. _____
4. _____
5. _____
6. _____
7. _____
8. _____
9. _____
10. _____
11. _____
12. _____
13. _____
14. _____
15. _____
16. _____
17. _____
18. _____
19. _____
20. _____
21. _____
22. _____
23. _____
24. _____
25. _____
26. _____
27. _____

PHYSICAL EXAMINATION CHECKLIST

1. _____
2. _____

3. ______________________________
4. ______________________________
5. ______________________________
6. ______________________________
7. ______________________________

Total DG Score ______ *Passing Score for DG is 24 points (70%)*

Examinee's Communication and Interpersonal Skills (CIS) Checklist

1. ______________________________
2. ______________________________
3. ______________________________
4. ______________________________
5. ______________________________
6. ______________________________
7. ______________________________
8. ______________________________
9. ______________________________
10. ______________________________
11. ______________________________
12. ______________________________
13. ______________________________
14. ______________________________
15. ______________________________
16. ______________________________
17. ______________________________
18. ______________________________
19. ______________________________
20. ______________________________

Total CIS Score ______ *Passing Score for CIS is 14 points (70%)*

123 Examinee's Spoken English Proficiency (SEP) Rating Scale

	Poor	Fair	Good	Very Good	Excellent
1. Ability of *patient* to understand *candidate*	1	2	3	4	5
2. Ability of *candidate* to understand *patient*	1	2	3	4	5
3. Candidate is articulate	1	2	3	4	5
4. Words are pronounced correctly	1	2	3	4	5
5. Range of vocabulary and sentence structure	1	2	3	4	5
6. Stress, rhythm, and intonation	1	2	3	4	5
7. Grammar	1	2	3	4	5
8. Repair strategies	1	2	3	4	5

Total SEP Score ______ *Passing Score for SEP is 28 points (70%)*

Examinee's Patient Note (PN)

HISTORY—Include any significant pertinent positives and negatives

PHYSICAL EXAMINATION— Include any significant pertinent positives and negatives

DIFFERENTIAL DIAGNOSIS

In order of likelihood, write no more than five (5) differential diagnoses

1.
2.
3.
4.
5.

DIAGNOSTIC WORKUP

Immediate plans, write no more than five (5) diagnostic studies

1.
2.
3.
4.
5.

Background Information for Standardized Patient

PATIENT BEHAVIOR
Shaking leg; shaking pen/pencil; looking at watch

AFFECT
Very professional; type A personality

PROVOCATIVE QUESTION(S) AND PLAUSIBLE ANSWER(S)
"How long is this going to take, because I have to get back to the office."

"We are going to do our very best to have you out of the clinic as quickly as possible, after we have done a thorough examination."

This patient wants to know the answer to what is going on, but she also doesn't want to know the answer—conflict! Be aware that sometimes it is seemingly more comforting for a patient to not know, than to confront the reality of what might be a significant degree of disease.

CHIEF COMPLAINT
"Loss of menstrual periods for 10 months"

HISTORY OF PRESENT ILLNESS
Susan Bell is a 31-year-old woman who comes for evaluation of loss of menstrual periods for the past 10 months. Ten months ago, she started to have irregular periods, and then 7 months ago, they stopped completely. At that time, she was not sexually active. About 5 months ago, she met Roger with whom she would like a lasting relationship and started having sex with him on a regular basis. She is now concerned whether or not she will ever be able to have children. Thinking that she might be pregnant, she did a home pregnancy test 1 month ago, which was negative. She has continued to have sexual relations since the test.

She has had a 10-pound weight gain in the past 6 months. She has noted some vaginal dryness in the past 2 months. She does not have hot flashes.

She denies headache, visual changes, hot/cold intolerance, diarrhea/constipation, or sleep problems.

PAST MEDICAL HISTORY
She had a pregnancy termination at age 23.

MEDICATIONS
None

ALLERGIES
None

SOCIAL HISTORY

She has a stressful job as the senior vice president of a large advertising firm. She was recently promoted to that position. It involves a good deal of responsibility. She does not smoke or use any recreational drugs.

FAMILY HISTORY

Her mother is alive and well at age 57. Her father, age 60, has multiple myeloma. She has one sister, age 33, who is fine.

SEXUAL HISTORY

She started having periods at age 12. Her LMP was 10 months ago. Prior to that, her periods occurred every 28 days for 5 days. Her last Pap smear was 1 year ago and was normal. She does not use any contraceptives.

REVIEW OF SYSTEMS

Noncontributory

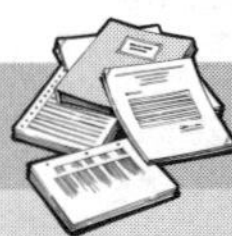

SP's Data Gathering (DG) Checklists

HISTORY CHECKLIST

1. I haven't had my periods for 10 months.
2. Ten months ago, my periods started to get irregular.
3. They stopped completely 7 months ago.
4. At that time, I wasn't sexually active.
5. I've been sexually active for the past 5 months.
6. I am concerned about whether I will ever be able to have children.
7. I thought that I might be pregnant.
8. I did a home pregnancy test 1 month ago. The test was negative.
9. I've had a 10-pound weight gain in the past 6 months.
10. I've noticed some vaginal dryness in the past 2 months.
11. I've never had hot flashes.
12. I do not have headaches.
13. I do not have any visual problems.
14. I have no hot/cold intolerance.
15. I do not have diarrhea or constipation.
16. I have no problems with sleep.
17. I had a pregnancy termination at age 23.
18. I do not take any medications.
19. I have no allergies.
20. I was recently promoted to senior vice president of a large advertising firm.
21. My job is very stressful.
22. I do not smoke or use any recreational drugs.
23. Neither my mother nor my sister has had anything like this.
24. I started having periods at age 12.
25. My periods occurred every 28 days for 5 days.
26. My last Pap smear was 1 year ago, and it was normal.
27. I do not use any contraceptives.

PHYSICAL CHECKLIST

1. Tested EOM's
2. Tested visual fields by confrontation field testing
3. Evaluated thyroid anteriorly and posteriorly

4. Evaluated heart by auscultation
5. Performed light palpation of the abdomen in all 4 quadrants *after* auscultation
6. Performed deep palpation of the abdomen in all 4 quadrants
7. Evaluated hands for tremor

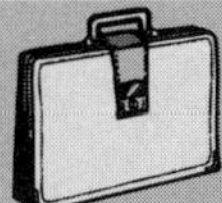

SP's Communication and Interpersonal Skills (CIS) Checklist

1. Knocked before entering
2. Opened interview by introducing self
3. Addressed patient using last name with introduction (e.g., Ms. Bell).
4. Appearance (e.g., clean and neat)
5. Allowed patient to express reason for seeking medical attention
6. Made comfortable eye contact
7. Did *not* use leading/biased questions (e.g., "You don't have…" or "You're not…")
8. Asked questions individually
9. Did *not* use the "Why" question
10. Concentrated and focused on patient's needs
11. Maintained comfortable and appropriate distance
12. Gave patient time to think and answer without interrupting
13. Used proper draping during physical exam
14. Did physical examination in an orderly manner
15. Summarized patient's condition (or asked patient to summarize)
16. Discussed diagnostic tests and/or next step in treatment in lay terms
17. Asked whether patient had other questions/concerns
18. Provided patient education/suggestions where appropriate
19. Did *not* give false assurances
20. Showed empathy

123 SP's Spoken English Proficiency (SEP) Rating Scale

	Poor	Fair	Good	Very Good	Excellent
1. Ability of *patient* to understand *candidate*	1	2	3	4	5
2. Ability of *candidate* to understand *patient*	1	2	3	4	5
3. Candidate is articulate	1	2	3	4	5
4. Words are pronounced correctly	1	2	3	4	5
5. Range of vocabulary and sentence structure	1	2	3	4	5
6. Stress, rhythm, and intonation	1	2	3	4	5
7. Grammar	1	2	3	4	5
8. Repair strategies	1	2	3	4	5

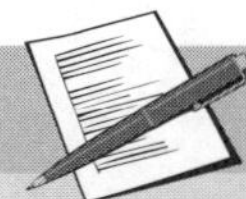

Example of a Satisfactory Patient Note (PN)

HISTORY—Include any significant pertinent positives and negatives

Ms. Susan Bell is a 31-year-old type A personality who presents with a chief complaint of "loss of menstrual periods for 10 months."

HISTORY OF PRESENT ILLNESS

- Periods became irregular 10 months ago and then stopped completely 7 months ago
- Not sexually active at that time
- Has been sexually active for the past 5 months
- Concerned now whether she will ever be able to have children
- Did a home pregnancy test 1 month ago which was negative
- (+) 10-pound weight gain in the past 6 months
- (+) vaginal dryness in the past 2 months
- (−) hot flashes, headaches, visual problems, hot/cold intolerance, diarrhea or constipation, problems with sleep

PAST MEDICAL HISTORY

- (+) pregnancy termination at age 23
- (−) medications
- (−) allergies

SOCIAL HISTORY

- Employed as the senior vice president of a large advertising firm
- Recently promoted; job very stressful
- (−) smoke or use any recreational drugs

FAMILY HISTORY

- (−) mother or sister have had similar problem

GYNECOLOGICAL

- Catamenia 12 × 28 × 5
- LMP 10 months ago
- Last Pap smear was 1 year ago and was normal
- (−) contraceptives

PHYSICAL EXAMINATION—Include any significant pertinent positives and negatives

GENERAL

- Physical examination reveals a well-developed, well-nourished, 31-year-old woman appearing her stated age.

VITAL SIGNS

- WNL

HEAD, EARS, EYES, NOSE, AND THROAT

- Eyes
  EOMs intact
  (−) visual field defects
- Thyroid
  (−) masses

CHEST

- Clear to P&A

HEART

- PMI 5th ICS-MCL
- (−) murmurs, gallops, or rubs

ABDOMEN

- (+) bowel sounds
- (−) tenderness
- (−) masses

EXTREMITIES

- (−) tremor

DIFFERENTIAL DIAGNOSIS

In order of likelihood, write no more than five (5) differential diagnoses

1. Pregnancy
2. Stress amenorrhea
3. Thyroid dysfunction
4. Premature ovarian failure
5. Polycystic ovary syndrome

DIAGNOSTIC WORKUP

Immediate plans, write no more than five (5) diagnostic studies

1. Pelvic and breast exams
2. CBC, LH, FSH, prolactin, TSH, free T_4, glucose, BUN, creatinine, testosterone, DHEAS
3. MRI of brain
4. Urine hCG
5. ______________________

CASE 22—Mr. Brian Rourke

Mr. Brian Rourke, a 53-year-old man, presents to the emergency room complaining of chest pain.

VITAL SIGNS

Temperature: 98.6° F	**Pulse:** 90 regular
Blood Pressure: 155/90	**Respiratory Rate:** 14 regular

EXAMINEE'S TASKS

In the next 15 minutes, you are to:

1. Take a focused history
2. Do a focused physical examination
3. Discuss your initial clinical impressions and workup plans with the patient
4. Write the Patient Note after leaving the room

Examinee's Data Gathering (DG) Checklists

HISTORY CHECKLIST

1. __________
2. __________
3. __________
4. __________
5. __________
6. __________
7. __________
8. __________
9. __________
10. __________
11. __________
12. __________
13. __________
14. __________
15. __________
16. __________
17. __________
18. __________
19. __________
20. __________

PHYSICAL EXAMINATION CHECKLIST

1. __________
2. __________
3. __________
4. __________
5. __________
6. __________

7. ______________________________

8. ______________________________

Total DG Score ______ *Passing Score for DG is 20 points (70%)*

Examinee's Communication and Interpersonal Skills (CIS) Checklist

1. ______________________________
2. ______________________________
3. ______________________________
4. ______________________________
5. ______________________________
6. ______________________________
7. ______________________________
8. ______________________________
9. ______________________________
10. ______________________________
11. ______________________________
12. ______________________________
13. ______________________________
14. ______________________________
15. ______________________________
16. ______________________________
17. ______________________________
18. ______________________________
19. ______________________________
20. ______________________________

Total CIS Score ______ *Passing Score for CIS is 14 points (70%)*

123 Examinee's Spoken English Proficiency (SEP) Rating Scale

	Poor	Fair	Good	Very Good	Excellent
1. Ability of *patient* to understand *candidate*	1	2	3	4	5
2. Ability of *candidate* to understand *patient*	1	2	3	4	5
3. Candidate is articulate	1	2	3	4	5
4. Words are pronounced correctly	1	2	3	4	5
5. Range of vocabulary and sentence structure	1	2	3	4	5
6. Stress, rhythm, and intonation	1	2	3	4	5
7. Grammar	1	2	3	4	5
8. Repair strategies	1	2	3	4	5

Total SEP Score _____ *Passing Score for SEP is 28 points (70%)*

Examinee's Patient Note (PN)

HISTORY—Include any significant pertinent positives and negatives

PHYSICAL EXAMINATION—Include any significant pertinent positives and negatives

DIFFERENTIAL DIAGNOSIS

In order of likelihood, write no more than five (5) differential diagnoses

1.
2.
3.
4.
5.

DIAGNOSTIC WORKUP

Immediate plans, write no more than five (5) diagnostic studies

1.
2.
3.
4.
5.

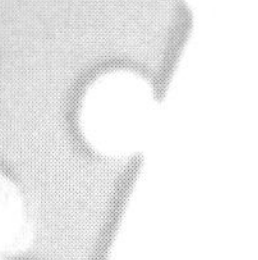

Remember that in each case you are taking care of the whole human being, not just a set of symptoms.

Background Information for Standardized Patient

PATIENT BEHAVIOR
Keeps his voice controlled; wants to be in control of himself and his emotions.

AFFECT
Scared; controlled panic

PROVOCATIVE QUESTION(S) AND PLAUSIBLE ANSWER(S)
"Doctor, am I going to die? Did I just have a heart attack?"

"I am going to take care of you and do everything possible."

CHIEF COMPLAINT
"I had a ton of bricks on my chest this morning"

HISTORY OF PRESENT ILLNESS
Brian Rourke is a 53-year-old man who was awakened this morning with the sudden onset of severe pressure in his chest that lasted 45 minutes. The pain was located in the center of his chest. He states that he also felt the pain in his left arm and back. He describes the pain as about an 8 out of 10. He rested in bed, and it finally went away, but he decided to come to the emergency room to be evaluated. He also had numbness in the fingers of both his hands. He also states that he had shortness of breath, nausea, one episode of vomiting, and sweating when he had the pain.

He has had similar, but not as severe, chest pain in the past 3 months. He saw his doctor, who recommended a stress test, but he refused to have the test because he was too scared. He now asks, "Was I stupid?" The other episodes of chest pain were associated with strenuous work and after a big meal.

PAST MEDICAL HISTORY
He has had high blood pressure, high cholesterol, and diabetes for more than 15 years and is on medications (see below).

MEDICATIONS
Atenolol 100 mg daily
Lisinopril 20 mg daily
Lipitor 20 mg daily
Hydrochlorothiazide 50 mg daily
Aspirin
Metformin 500 mg twice daily

ALLERGIES
Shellfish (rash)

SOCIAL HISTORY

He is a financial advisor working in a consulting firm. It's a very-high-pressure job. He doesn't drink alcohol. He has never used recreational drugs. He smokes 1 ppd × 20 years. He is divorced and is living with his new girlfriend for the past 2 years. He has no children.

FAMILY HISTORY

His mother is 75 years old and has diabetes and macular degeneration. His father died of a heart attack 6 years ago at the age of 69. His brother, who is now 58, had a heart attack 2 years ago.

SEXUAL HISTORY

He was sexually active with his girlfriend until 3 months ago when his symptoms started. He's now afraid to have sexual relations.

REVIEW OF SYSTEMS

Noncontributory

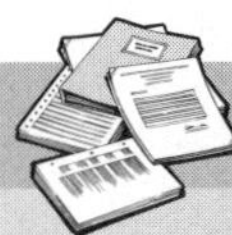

SP's Data Gathering (DG) Checklists

HISTORY CHECKLIST

1. I had a ton of bricks on my chest this morning.
2. I awakened this morning with the sudden onset of severe pressure in my chest that lasted 45 minutes.
3. The pain was located in the center of my chest.
4. I also felt the pain in my left arm and back.
5. The pain was about an 8 out of 10.
6. I rested in bed, and it finally went away.
7. I had numbness in the fingers of both my hands.
8. I had shortness of breath, nausea, one episode of vomiting, and sweating when I had the pain. *(at least two)*
9. I had similar, but not as severe, chest pain in the past 3 months.
10. I saw my doctor, who recommended a stress test, but I refused because I was too scared.
11. The other episodes of chest pain were associated with strenuous work and after a big meal.
12. I have had high blood pressure for 15 years.
13. I have high cholesterol for about 15 years.
14. I have had diabetes for more than 15 years.
15. I take atenolol 100 mg, lisinopril 20 mg, Lipitor 20 mg, hydrochlorothiazide 50 mg, aspirin daily; I take metformin 500 mg twice daily.
16. I am allergic to shellfish.
17. I've been smoking 1 ppd cigarettes × 20 years.
18. My father died of a heart attack 6 years ago at the age of 69.
19. My brother had a heart attack 2 years ago.
20. I'm now afraid to have sex with my girlfriend.

PHYSICAL CHECKLIST

1. Took blood pressure both upper extremities
2. Performed ophthalmoscopic examination
3. Palpated carotids after auscultation
4. Performed auscultation of the lungs
5. Performed auscultation of the heart
6. Performed light palpation of the abdomen in all 4 quadrants *after* auscultation
7. Evaluated liver size by palpation
8. Evaluated lower extremities for edema

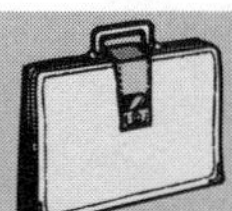

SP's Communication and Interpersonal Skills (CIS) Checklist

1. Knocked before entering
2. Opened interview by introducing self
3. Addressed patient using last name with introduction (e.g., Mr. Rourke)
4. Appearance (e.g., clean and neat)
5. Allowed patient to express reason for seeking medical attention
6. Made comfortable eye contact
7. Did *not* use leading/biased questions (e.g., "You don't have…" or "You're not…")
8. Asked questions individually
9. Did *not* use the "Why" question
10. Concentrated and focused on patient's needs
11. Maintained comfortable and appropriate distance
12. Gave patient time to think and answer without interrupting
13. Used proper draping during physical exam
14. Did physical examination in an orderly manner
15. Summarized patient's condition (or asked patient to summarize)
16. Discussed diagnostic tests and/or next step in treatment in lay terms
17. Asked whether patient had other questions/concerns
18. Provided patient education/suggestions where appropriate
19. Did *not* give false reassurances
20. Showed empathy

123 SP's Spoken English Proficiency (SEP) Rating Scale

	Poor	Fair	Good	Very Good	Excellent
1. Ability of *patient* to understand *candidate*	1	2	3	4	5
2. Ability of *candidate* to understand *patient*	1	2	3	4	5
3. Candidate is articulate	1	2	3	4	5
4. Words are pronounced correctly	1	2	3	4	5
5. Range of vocabulary and sentence structure	1	2	3	4	5
6. Stress, rhythm, and intonation	1	2	3	4	5
7. Grammar	1	2	3	4	5
8. Repair strategies	1	2	3	4	5

Example of a Satisfactory Patient Note (PN)

HISTORY—Include any significant pertinent positives and negatives

Mr. Brian Rourke is a 53-year-old who presents to the ER with the chief complaint of "I had a ton of bricks on my chest this morning."

HISTORY OF PRESENT ILLNESS

- Awoke this morning with the sudden onset of severe pressure in chest that lasted 45 minutes
- Pain was located in the center of his chest and in left arm and back
- Pain was about an 8 out of 10
- Relieved by resting in bed
- (+) numbness in the fingers of both hands
- (+) shortness of breath, nausea, one episode of vomiting, and sweating with the pain
- Similar, but not as severe, chest pain in the past 3 months
- Saw doctor who recommended a stress test, but patient refused because he was too scared
- Other episodes of chest pain associated with strenuous work and after a big meal
- (+) high blood pressure, high cholesterol, diabetes for more than 15 years

PAST MEDICAL HISTORY

- Medications
  Atenolol 100 mg daily
  Lisinopril 20 mg daily
  Lipitor 20 mg daily
  Hydrochlorothiazide 50 mg daily
  Aspirin daily
  Metformin 500 mg twice daily
- (+) allergy—shellfish

SOCIAL HISTORY

- Financial advisor—stressful job
- Divorced, no children
- Lives with girlfriend × 2 years
- (+) smoking—1 ppd cigarettes × 20 years
- (–) recreational drug use

FAMILY HISTORY

- Mother—75 years old, diabetes, macular degeneration
- Father died—MI, age 69
- Brother—MI, age 56

SEXUAL HISTORY

- Sexually active with his girlfriend until 3 months ago when his symptoms started; now afraid to have sex

PHYSICAL EXAMINATION—Include any significant pertinent positives and negatives

GENERAL

- Physical examination reveals a well-developed, slightly obese, 53-year-old man appearing his stated age and in moderate distress, complaining of chest pain

VITAL SIGNS

- BP (RA) 155/90; (LA) 150/90
- Otherwise WNL

HEAD, EARS, EYES, NOSE, AND THROAT

- Carotids (–) bruit, normal contour
- Optic discs clear with sharp disc margins; color WNL; vasculature WNL

CHEST

- Clear to P&A

CARDIAC

- PMI 5th ICS-MCL
- S_1S_2 WNL
- (+) S_4
- (–) murmurs or rubs

ABDOMEN

- (+) BS
- (–) tenderness, masses
- (–) hepatosplenomegaly

EXTREMITIES

- (–) edema present

DIFFERENTIAL DIAGNOSIS

In order of likelihood, write no more than five (5) differential diagnoses

1. Coronary artery disease (R/O MI, ischemia)
2. R/O aortic dissection
3. R/O GERD
4. R/O Pericarditis
5. R/O Costochondritis

DIAGNOSTIC WORKUP

Immediate plans, write no more than five (5) diagnostic studies

1. Serial ECGs
2. CBC, CPK, CPK-MB, troponin, lipid profile
3. Chest x-ray
4. Transthoracic echocardiogram
5. Cardiac catheterization

CASE 23—Mr. Thomas McMann

Mr. Thomas McMann, a 58-year-old man, presents to clinic complaining of loss of energy.

VITAL SIGNS

Temperature: 98.6° F	**Pulse:** 80 regular
Blood Pressure: 130/70	**Respiratory Rate:** 12 regular

EXAMINEE'S TASKS

In the next 15 minutes, you are to:

1. Take a focused history
2. Do a focused physical examination
3. Discuss your initial clinical impressions and workup plans with the patient
4. Write the Patient Note after leaving the room

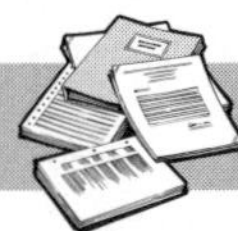

Examinee's Data Gathering (DG) Checklists

HISTORY CHECKLIST

1. _____
2. _____
3. _____
4. _____
5. _____
6. _____
7. _____
8. _____
9. _____
10. _____
11. _____
12. _____
13. _____
14. _____
15. _____
16. _____
17. _____
18. _____
19. _____
20. _____
21. _____
22. _____

PHYSICAL EXAMINATION CHECKLIST

1. _____
2. _____
3. _____
4. _____
5. _____

6. ______________________________
7. ______________________________
8. ______________________________

Total DG Score ______ *Passing Score for DG is 21 points (70%)*

Examinee's Communication and Interpersonal Skills (CIS) Checklist

1. ______________________________
2. ______________________________
3. ______________________________
4. ______________________________
5. ______________________________
6. ______________________________
7. ______________________________
8. ______________________________
9. ______________________________
10. ______________________________
11. ______________________________
12. ______________________________
13. ______________________________
14. ______________________________
15. ______________________________
16. ______________________________
17. ______________________________
18. ______________________________
19. ______________________________
20. ______________________________

Total CIS Score ______ *Passing Score for CIS is 14 points (70%)*

123 Examinee's Spoken English Proficiency (SEP) Rating Scale

	Poor	Fair	Good	Very Good	Excellent
1. Ability of *patient* to understand *candidate*	1	2	3	4	5
2. Ability of *candidate* to understand *patient*	1	2	3	4	5
3. Candidate is articulate	1	2	3	4	5
4. Words are pronounced correctly	1	2	3	4	5
5. Range of vocabulary and sentence structure	1	2	3	4	5
6. Stress, rhythm, and intonation	1	2	3	4	5
7. Grammar	1	2	3	4	5
8. Repair strategies	1	2	3	4	5

Total SEP Score ______ *Passing Score for SEP is 28 points (70%)*

Examinee's Patient Note (PN)

HISTORY—Include any significant pertinent positives and negatives

PHYSICAL EXAMINATION—Include any significant pertinent positives and negatives

DIFFERENTIAL DIAGNOSIS

In order of likelihood, write no more than five (5) differential diagnoses

1.
2.
3.
4.
5.

DIAGNOSTIC WORKUP

Immediate plans, write no more than five (5) diagnostic studies

1.
2.
3.
4.
5.

Only after the patient has told his/her story can the interviewer begin to put the puzzle together by using targeted direct questions.

Background Information for Standardized Patient

PATIENT BEHAVIOR

Moves as little as possible; sighs; even talking seems like an effort; yawns

AFFECT

Sad; down

PROVOCATIVE QUESTION(S) AND PLAUSIBLE ANSWER(S)

"Will I ever feel better doc?"

"I can understand your concern. Let's get some more information first."

"Do I have cancer?"

"We need to perform a physical examination and do some laboratory tests. When we get the results, I'll be in a better position to answer your question."

CHIEF COMPLAINT

"I don't have any energy any more. I'm tired all the time."

HISTORY OF PRESENT ILLNESS

Thomas McMann is a 58-year-old man who comes for evaluation of loss of energy. For the past 6 weeks, he has become very tired in the afternoons around 3 PM. He sleeps well and has no trouble falling asleep and gets up at his regular time of 6 AM. He does not snore, and his wife has not noticed any change in his sleeping pattern.

He has noticed that in the past 2 months he gets up about twice every night to urinate. Although he seems to be eating normally, and even snacking more than previously, he has lost about 7 pounds in the past 2 months. He also notes that he has been drinking more, especially fruit juices.

He has no history of tremor, hot/cold intolerance, palpitations, mood changes, hair changes.

PAST MEDICAL HISTORY

He has had high blood pressure for about 15 years, which is well controlled using medications.

MEDICATIONS

Lisinopril 20 mg daily
Aspirin

ALLERGIES

Penicillin (rash)

SOCIAL HISTORY

He is the senior accountant for a large law firm. He is happily married with five children, ages 25 to 33. They are all well. He has two grandchildren. He drinks "socially" on weekends. He tried marijuana in college, but he has not used it since. He does not use any other recreational drug.

FAMILY HISTORY

His father is 82 and had a heart attack several years ago. He has high blood pressure. His mother is 81 and has diabetes. His sister, age 56, has some type of thyroid disease.

SEXUAL HISTORY

He is sexually active with only his wife. In the past 6 weeks, he has not had any sexual relations because he has been so tired.

REVIEW OF SYSTEMS

He's had blurry vision for the past 2–3 months. He saw his ophthalmologist a month ago for new glasses, but he thinks his vision is still blurry. He noted last month that he developed some "pins and needles" sensation in his feet.

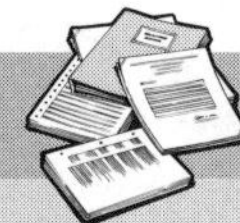

SP's Data Gathering (DG) Checklists

HISTORY CHECKLIST

1. I don't have any energy any more. I'm tired all the time.
2. For the past 6 weeks, I have become very tired in the afternoons around 3 PM.
3. I sleep well and have no trouble falling asleep.
4. I get up at my regular time of 6 AM.
5. I do not snore.
6. My wife has not noticed any change in my sleeping pattern.
7. I noticed that in the past 2 months, I have to get up about twice a night to urinate.
8. I have lost about 7 pounds in the past 2 months.
9. I eat normally and am even snacking more than previously.
10. I've been drinking more lately, especially fruit juices.
11. I don't have a tremor.
12. I do not have hot/cold intolerance.
13. I do not have palpitations.
14. I do not have any mood changes.
15. I haven't noticed any hair changes.
16. I've had high blood pressure for about 15 years.
17. I take lisinopril 20 mg and aspirin daily.
18. I am allergic to penicillin; I get a rash.
19. My mother is 81 years old and has diabetes.
20. My sister is 56 years old and has some type of thyroid disease.
21. I've had blurry vision for the past 2–3 months.
22. In the past month, I've had a "pins and needles" sensation in my feet.

PHYSICAL CHECKLIST

1. Took blood pressure
2. Evaluated for orthostatic hypotension
3. Performed ophthalmoscopic examination
4. Palpated thyroid (anteriorly and posteriorly)
5. Performed auscultation of lung fields
6. Performed light palpation of the abdomen in all 4 quadrants *after* auscultation
7. Performed deep palpation of the abdomen in all 4 quadrants
8. Evaluated liver by palpation

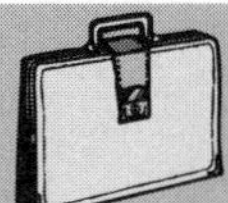

SP's Communication and Interpersonal Skills (CIS) Checklist

1. Knocked before entering
2. Opened interview by introducing self
3. Addressed patient using last name with introduction (e.g., Mr. McMann)
4. Appearance (e.g., clean and neat)
5. Allowed patient to express reason for seeking medical attention
6. Made comfortable eye contact
7. Did *not* use leading/biased questions (e.g., "You don't have…" or "You're not…")
8. Asked questions individually
9. Did *not* use the "Why" question
10. Concentrated and focused on patient's needs
11. Maintained comfortable and appropriate distance
12. Gave patient time to think and answer without interrupting
13. Used proper draping during physical exam
14. Did physical examination in an orderly manner
15. Summarized patient's condition (or asked patient to summarize)
16. Discussed diagnostic tests and/or next step in treatment in lay terms
17. Asked whether patient had other questions/concerns
18. Provided patient education/suggestions where appropriate
19. Did *not* give false assurances
20. Showed empathy

123 SP's Spoken English Proficiency (SEP) Rating Scale

	Poor	Fair	Good	Very Good	Excellent
1. Ability of *patient* to understand *candidate*	1	2	3	4	5
2. Ability of *candidate* to understand *patient*	1	2	3	4	5
3. Candidate is articulate	1	2	3	4	5
4. Words are pronounced correctly	1	2	3	4	5
5. Range of vocabulary and sentence structure	1	2	3	4	5
6. Stress, rhythm, and intonation	1	2	3	4	5
7. Grammar	1	2	3	4	5
8. Repair strategies	1	2	3	4	5

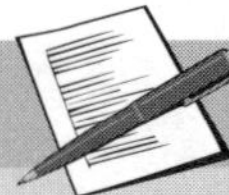

Example of a Satisfactory Patient Note (PN)

HISTORY—Include any significant pertinent positives and negatives

Mr. Thomas McMann is a 58-year-old man who presents to clinic with the chief complaint of "I don't have any energy any more. I'm tired all the time."

HISTORY OF PRESENT ILLNESS

- Tired in the afternoons around 3 PM for the past 6 weeks
- Sleeps well and has no trouble falling asleep; gets up at his regular time of 6 AM
- Does not snore
- No change in sleeping pattern
- Nocturia × 2 for past 2 months
- (+) 7-pound weight loss in past 2 months despite eating normally and snacking more
- (+) drinking more lately, especially fruit juices
- (–) tremor, hot/cold intolerance, palpitations, mood changes, or hair changes

PAST MEDICAL HISTORY

- (+) HT × 15 years
- Medications
  Lisinopril 20 mg daily
  Aspirin daily
- (+) Allergies—PCN (rash)

SOCIAL HISTORY

- Senior accountant in a law firm
- Married, 5 children, ages 25–33
- Drinks "socially" on weekends
- (–) recreational drug use

FAMILY HISTORY

- Mother—81 years old, diabetes
- Father—82 years old—CAD, HT
- Sister, age 56—thyroid disease

REVIEW OF SYSTEMS

- (+) blurry vision for 2–3 months
- (+) "pins and needles" sensation in feet

PHYSICAL EXAMINATION—Include any significant pertinent positives and negatives

GENERAL

- Physical examination reveals a well-developed, slightly thin, 58-year-old man appearing his stated age and in no acute distress.

VITAL SIGNS

- BP 130/70
- (–) orthostatic changes
- Otherwise WNL

HEAD, EARS, EYES, NOSE, AND THROAT

- PERRL
- Optic discs clear with sharp disc margins; color WNL; vasculature WNL
- Thyroid (–) masses or bruits

CHEST

- Clear to P&A

ABDOMEN

- (+) BS
- (–) tenderness, masses
- (–) hepatomegaly

DIFFERENTIAL DIAGNOSIS

In order of likelihood, write no more than five (5) differential diagnoses

1. Diabetes mellitus
2. Hyperthyroidism
3. R/O occult cancer (e.g., colon, lung, pancreas)
4. ______________________________
5. ______________________________

DIAGNOSTIC WORKUP

Immediate plans, write no more than five (5) diagnostic studies

1. Rectal exam and stool for FOBT
2. CBC, fasting glucose, TSH, T_4, PSA
3. Colonoscopy
4. CT of abdomen
5. Chest x-ray

CASE 24—Ms. Eva Marchevska

Ms. Eva Marchevska, an 87-year-old woman, presents to clinic complaining of difficulty in sleeping and fatigue.

VITAL SIGNS

Temperature: 98.6° F	**Pulse:** 85 regular
Blood Pressure: 155/70	**Respiratory Rate:** 14 regular

EXAMINEE'S TASKS

In the next 15 minutes, you are to:

1. Take a focused history
2. Do a focused physical examination
3. Discuss your initial clinical impressions and workup plans with the patient
4. Write the Patient Note after leaving the room

Examinee's Data Gathering (DG) Checklists

HISTORY CHECKLIST

1. ______
2. ______
3. ______
4. ______
5. ______
6. ______
7. ______
8. ______
9. ______
10. ______
11. ______
12. ______
13. ______
14. ______
15. ______
16. ______
17. ______
18. ______
19. ______
20. ______

PHYSICAL EXAMINATION CHECKLIST

1. ______
2. ______
3. ______
4. ______
5. ______
6. ______

7. ____________________
8. ____________________

Total DG Score ______ *Passing Score for DG is 20 points (70%)*

Examinee's Communication and Interpersonal Skills (CIS) Checklist

1. ____________________
2. ____________________
3. ____________________
4. ____________________
5. ____________________
6. ____________________
7. ____________________
8. ____________________
9. ____________________
10. ____________________
11. ____________________
12. ____________________
13. ____________________
14. ____________________
15. ____________________
16. ____________________
17. ____________________
18. ____________________
19. ____________________
20. ____________________

Total CIS Score ______ *Passing Score for CIS is 14 points (70%)*

123 Examinee's Spoken English Proficiency (SEP) Rating Scale

	Poor	Fair	Good	Very Good	Excellent
1. Ability of *patient* to understand *candidate*	1	2	3	4	5
2. Ability of *candidate* to understand *patient*	1	2	3	4	5
3. Candidate is articulate	1	2	3	4	5
4. Words are pronounced correctly	1	2	3	4	5
5. Range of vocabulary and sentence structure	1	2	3	4	5
6. Stress, rhythm, and intonation	1	2	3	4	5
7. Grammar	1	2	3	4	5
8. Repair strategies	1	2	3	4	5

Total SEP Score ______ *Passing Score for SEP is 28 points (70%)*

Examinee's Patient Note (PN)

HISTORY—Include any significant pertinent positives and negatives

PHYSICAL EXAMINATION— Include any significant pertinent positives and negatives

DIFFERENTIAL DIAGNOSIS

In order of likelihood, write no more than five (5) differential diagnoses

1.
2.
3.
4.
5.

DIAGNOSTIC WORKUP

Immediate plans, write no more than five (5) diagnostic studies

1.
2.
3.
4.
5.

Background Information for Standardized Patient

PATIENT BEHAVIOR

Lethargic; doesn't look much at the interviewer; doesn't move very much; many monosyllabic answers

AFFECT

Depressed; looks sad

PROVOCATIVE QUESTION(S) AND PLAUSIBLE ANSWER(S)

"I didn't even want to come here today, but my daughter insisted. What's the point?"

"It is good that you came in, and we are going to try to get to the bottom of why you are not feeling like yourself."

ADDITIONAL NOTES

She has a lot of guilt about leaving her mother the day the Warsaw Ghetto was burned and doesn't talk much about it unless the examiner shows much empathy.

CHIEF COMPLAINT

"I can't sleep and I'm always tired."

HISTORY OF PRESENT ILLNESS

Eva Marchevska is an 87-year-old woman who comes to clinic with the complaint of insomnia and fatigue for the past year. She came today on the insistence from her 58-year-old daughter.

She describes that she has no problem falling asleep after the 11 PM news, but she awakens at about 3 AM. She relates that she has terrible recurring nightmares and flashbacks about her experience during the Holocaust when she was in Poland. Her entire first family was killed, and she feels much guilt about leaving her mother the day the Warsaw Ghetto was burned. She has had a 10-pound weight loss in the past 4 months and a poor appetite. She also has had a dull ache in her midback for the past 2–3 months. Nothing seems to make it better or worse. She describes it as a 5 out of 10 in severity. It does not seem to be felt in any other area of her body except the middle of her back. There is no relation between the pain and eating. She has not had nausea, vomiting, or diarrhea, or blood in her stools. She tries to remain active, but the fatigue seems to be getting worse. She has lost interest in many things that previously made her happy. She has no suicidal ideations or plans. Her only granddaughter, age 28, is getting married in a few months, and she just can't get happy over it.

Remember that in all patients older than age 65 years, some portions of a mini-mental exam must be administered early in the encounter to ensure that the person is oriented to person, time, and place. Otherwise, the entire interview may be invalid. Also notice that the interviewer said that he/she was going to "try" to get to the bottom of the problem; sometimes you cannot determine a diagnosis at that point in time!

PAST MEDICAL HISTORY

She had a cholecystectomy about 50 years ago. She has a 20-year history of high blood pressure, which is controlled by medications.

MEDICATIONS

Norvasc 5 mg daily
Hydrochlorothiazide 50 mg daily

ALLERGIES

None

SOCIAL HISTORY

She is a housewife. She is a survivor of World War II. She was living in Warsaw when the war broke out. She was married with a 1-year-old son; both her husband and son were killed, as were her parents and sister, during the war. Her second husband died suddenly 3 days after a routine prostatectomy about 20 years ago. She has one daughter, age 58, and one granddaughter, age 28. She smoked 4–5 cigarettes a day for many years but stopped about 40 years ago. She doesn't drink alcohol or use any other recreational drug.

FAMILY HISTORY

See Social History

SEXUAL HISTORY

She has not been sexually active for many years.

REVIEW OF SYSTEMS

Noncontributory

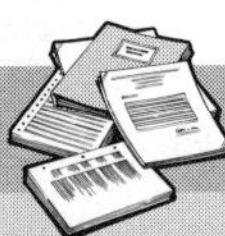

SP's Data Gathering (DG) Checklists

HISTORY CHECKLIST

1. I can't sleep, and I'm always tired.
2. I had this for about a year.
3. My daughter insisted that I come to see you today.
4. I have no problem falling asleep, but I get up very early, at about 3 AM.
5. I have terrible nightmares.
6. My entire first family was killed in Poland.
7. I've lost about 10 pounds in the past 4 months.
8. I don't seem to have an appetite any more.
9. I have had a dull ache in my midback for the past 2–3 months.
10. Nothing seems to make my back pain better or worse.
11. I guess the pain is about a 5 out of 10 in severity.
12. I don't feel the pain in any other area of my body except the middle of back.
13. There is no relation between the pain and eating.
14. I have not had nausea or vomiting.
15. I don't have diarrhea.
16. There is no blood in my stools.
17. I try to remain active, but the fatigue seems to be getting worse.
18. I have lost interest in so many things that previously made me happy.
19. I don't want to hurt myself.
20. I take Norvasc 5 mg daily and hydrochlorothiazide 50 mg daily for high blood pressure.

PHYSICAL CHECKLIST

1. Took blood pressure
2. Evaluated thyroid by palpation, anteriorly and posteriorly
3. Evaluated lung fields by auscultation
4. Evaluated the heart by auscultation
5. Performed light palpation of the abdomen in all 4 quadrants *after* auscultation
6. Performed deep palpation of the abdomen in all 4 quadrants
7. Evaluated liver by palpation
8. Checked orientation to person, place, and time

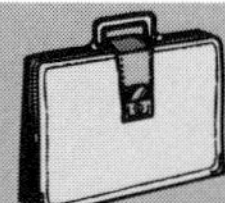

SP's Communication and Interpersonal Skills (CIS) Checklist

1. Knocked before entering
2. Opened interview by introducing self
3. Addressed patient using last name with introduction (e.g., Ms. Marchevska)
4. Appearance (e.g., clean and neat)
5. Allowed patient to express reason for seeking medical attention
6. Made comfortable eye contact
7. Did *not* use leading/biased questions (e.g., "You don't have…" or "You're not…")
8. Asked questions individually
9. Did *not* use the "Why" question
10. Concentrated and focused on patient's needs
11. Maintained comfortable and appropriate distance
12. Gave patient time to think and answer without interrupting
13. Used proper draping during physical exam
14. Did physical examination in an orderly manner
15. Summarized patient's condition (or asked patient to summarize)
16. Discussed diagnostic tests and/or next step in treatment in lay terms
17. Asked whether patient had other questions/concerns
18. Provided patient education/suggestions where appropriate
19. Did *not* give false assurances
20. Showed empathy

123 SP's Spoken English Proficiency (SEP) Rating Scale

	Poor	Fair	Good	Very Good	Excellent
1. Ability of *patient* to understand *candidate*	1	2	3	4	5
2. Ability of *candidate* to understand *patient*	1	2	3	4	5
3. Candidate is articulate	1	2	3	4	5
4. Words are pronounced correctly	1	2	3	4	5
5. Range of vocabulary and sentence structure	1	2	3	4	5
6. Stress, rhythm, and intonation	1	2	3	4	5
7. Grammar	1	2	3	4	5
8. Repair strategies	1	2	3	4	5

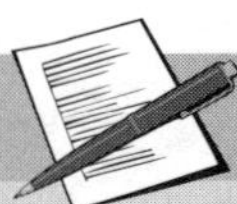

Example of a Satisfactory Patient Note (PN)

HISTORY—Include any significant pertinent positives and negatives

Ms. Eva Marchevska is an 87-year-old Holocaust survivor who presents now to clinic with the chief complaint of "I can't sleep and I'm always tired" for the past year. She came today at the insistence of her daughter.

HISTORY OF PRESENT ILLNESS

- No problem falling asleep but awakens early at about 3 AM
- c/o terrible recurring nightmares about the Holocaust; entire first family killed
- (+) 10-pound weight loss in the past 4 months associated with decreased appetite
- c/o dull ache in midback for past 2–3 months; nothing seems to make it better or worse
- Pain described as a 5 out of 10 in severity; no radiation; no relation to eating
- (−) nausea, vomiting, diarrhea, and blood in stools
- Fatigue seems to be getting worse
- Loss of interest in things that previously made her happy
- No suicidal ideations

PAST MEDICAL HISTORY

- (+) cholecystectomy—50 years ago
- (+) HT × 20 years
- Medications
  Norvasc 5 mg daily
  Hydrochlorothiazide 50 mg daily
- (−) allergies

SOCIAL HISTORY

- Housewife, widow
- Survivor of World War II
- Living in Warsaw when the war broke out; married with a 1-year-old son; both husband and son killed, as were her parents and sister, during the war
- Second husband died suddenly 3 days after routine prostatectomy 20 years ago
- One daughter, age 58, and one granddaughter, age 28
- Smoked 4–5 cigarettes a day for many years but stopped about 40 years ago
- (−) alcohol or other recreational drugs

FAMILY HISTORY

- See Social History

PHYSICAL EXAMINATION—Include any significant pertinent positives and negatives

GENERAL

- Physical examination reveals a well-developed, thin, 87-year-old woman appearing her stated age, complaining of difficulty in sleeping and fatigue and looking depressed

VITAL SIGNS

- BP 155/70
- Otherwise WNL

HEAD, EARS, EYES, NOSE, AND THROAT

- Optic discs clear with sharp disc margins; color WNL; vasculature WNL
- Thyroid (–) masses or bruit

CHEST

- Clear to P&A

CARDIAC

- PMI 5th ICS-MCL
- S_1S_2 WNL
- (–) murmurs, gallops, or rubs

ABDOMEN

- (+) BS
- (–) tenderness, masses
- (–) hepatomegaly

NEUROLOGICAL

- Oriented × 3
- No cognitive impairment (able to remember 3 objects, spell "earth" forward and backward, and follow 3 commands)

DIFFERENTIAL DIAGNOSIS

In order of likelihood, write no more than five (5) differential diagnoses

1. Major depression
2. Post-traumatic stress syndrome
3. Anxiety disorder
4. Pancreatic carcinoma
5. Hypothyroidism

DIAGNOSTIC WORKUP

Immediate plans, write no more than five (5) diagnostic studies

1. Rectal exam and stool for FOBT
2. CBC, amylase, lipase, AST, ALT, bilirubin, alkaline phosphatase, TSH, CEA, CA 27-29, glucose
3. CT of abdomen
4. Upper endoscopy
5. Upper GI series

CASE 25—Mr. Jacques Milano

Mr. Jacques Milano, a 17-year-old man, presents to you in clinic complaining of "feeling down." His football coach wants him to be evaluated by you.

VITAL SIGNS

Temperature: 98.6° F	**Pulse:** 80 regular
Blood Pressure: 135/85	**Respiratory Rate:** 12 regular

EXAMINEE'S TASKS

In the next 15 minutes, you are to:

1) Take a focused history
2) Do a focused physical examination
3) Discuss your initial clinical impressions and workup plans with the patient
4) Write the Patient Note after leaving the room

Examinee's Data Gathering (DG) Checklists

HISTORY CHECKLIST

1. ______
2. ______
3. ______
4. ______
5. ______
6. ______
7. ______
8. ______
9. ______
10. ______
11. ______
12. ______
13. ______
14. ______
15. ______
16. ______
17. ______
18. ______
19. ______
20. ______
21. ______

PHYSICAL EXAMINATION CHECKLIST

1. ______
2. ______
3. ______
4. ______
5. ______
6. ______

Total DG Score ______ *Passing Score for DG is 19 points (70%)*

Examinee's Communication and Interpersonal Skills (CIS) Checklist

1. ______
2. ______
3. ______
4. ______
5. ______
6. ______
7. ______
8. ______
9. ______
10. ______
11. ______
12. ______
13. ______
14. ______
15. ______
16. ______
17. ______
18. ______
19. ______
20. ______

Total CIS Score ______ *Passing Score for CIS is 14 points (70%)*

123 Examinee's Spoken English Proficiency (SEP) Rating Scale

	Poor	Fair	Good	Very Good	Excellent
1. Ability of *patient* to understand *candidate*	1	2	3	4	5
2. Ability of *candidate* to understand *patient*	1	2	3	4	5
3. Candidate is articulate	1	2	3	4	5
4. Words are pronounced correctly	1	2	3	4	5
5. Range of vocabulary and sentence structure	1	2	3	4	5
6. Stress, rhythm, and intonation	1	2	3	4	5
7. Grammar	1	2	3	4	5
8. Repair strategies	1	2	3	4	5

Total SEP Score ______ *Passing Score for SEP is 28 points (70%)*

Examinee's Patient Note (PN)

HISTORY— Include any significant pertinent positives and negatives from the history

PHYSICAL EXAMINATION—Include any significant pertinent positives and negatives from the physical examination

DIFFERENTIAL DIAGNOSIS

In order of likelihood, write no more than five (5) differential diagnoses

1.
2.
3.
4.
5.

DIAGNOSTIC WORKUP

Immediate plans, write no more than five (5) diagnostic studies

1.
2.
3.
4.
5.

In interviewing an adolescent, it is important to establish confidentiality; assure the patient that what he/she discloses will remain private.

Background Information for Standardized Patient

PATIENT BEHAVIOR

Doesn't meet the doctor's eyes; not too forthcoming with verbal responses

AFFECT

Bored; listless; sullen

PROVOCATIVE QUESTION(S) AND PLAUSIBLE ANSWER(S)

"When can I leave?"

"I want to help you feel better. It's good that your coach encouraged you to come in. As soon as I have completed the history and physical examination, we can discuss it further. It will not take too long."

CHIEF COMPLAINT

"I'm feeling down."

HISTORY OF PRESENT ILLNESS

Jacques Milano is a 17-year-old high school senior who has been "feeling down" for the past few months. He came in today at the insistence of his football coach. Life was fine up to about 10 months ago when his father died suddenly at the age of 43 from a heart attack. He had been very close to him. His grades have been slipping at school also. He used to get mostly B's, but now he's been getting C's and even a few D's because of a lack of interest. He has noticed that he has been awakening at 4 AM recently and cannot get back to sleep. He goes to sleep about midnight. For the past 8 months, he's also noticed that he just cannot concentrate on anything. He has even considered suicide, but he has no plan.

PAST MEDICAL HISTORY

He's been healthy all his life. He has been playing football in high school for 3 years. For the past 3 years, he has also been lifting weights, running, and biking to build up his muscles. For the past 2 years, he's been taking steroids to build up the bulk of his muscles. He takes them in cycles (2 months on, 2 months off). During the football season, he stops taking them because of routine blood checks.

MEDICATIONS

Steroids as indicated above

ALLERGIES

Penicillin (rash)

SOCIAL HISTORY

Because of "feeling down" and his poor grades in school, he started snorting cocaine about 5 months ago. He uses about 3/4 to 1 gram per week. It seems to make him feel better. He admits to drinking 3–4 cans of beer on the weekends; he denies smoking.

FAMILY HISTORY

He lives at home with his mother (whom, he feels, doesn't understand him) and his two siblings: a sister Monique, age 16, and a brother Louis, age 15. They live in a home in a suburban area in the Northeast. No one at home knows about his drug use. He has been recruited by seven colleges for sports scholarships but is worried that his grades are now so bad, they may reject him.

SEXUAL HISTORY

He has been sexually active since he was 14. He denies having had any sexually transmitted disease. He uses condoms. He's had about five girlfriends and slept with four of them. Over the past 3 months, he's had trouble maintaining an erection, and he is embarrassed by not being able to perform sexually. He is currently not in any relationship, which also bothers him.

REVIEW OF SYSTEMS

He's recently noticed an increase in acne on his face, chest, and back.

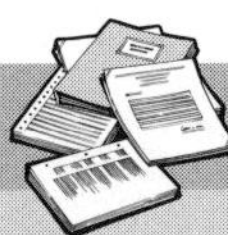

SP's Data Gathering (DG) Checklists

HISTORY CHECKLIST

1. My football coach wanted me to come in today.
2. I am a senior in high school.
3. I live at home with my mother, sister, and brother.
4. I have one sister (age 16) and one brother (age 15).
5. I love football and play the end on the team.
6. I'm being recruited by 7 colleges on sports scholarships.
7. I've been working really hard weight-lifting for the past 3 years
8. Over the past 10 months, I've been feeling really down.
9. My father died suddenly from a heart attack 10 months ago.
10. My grades are slipping; I used to get mostly B's, but now it's mostly C's and even some D's.
11. I've been getting up real early, about 4 AM, and can't get back to sleep.
12. I can't seem to concentrate on anything for the past 8 months.
13. I have some thoughts about suicide.
14. I've noticed a lot of acne on my face, chest, and back recently.
15. I started using cocaine about 5 months ago; it seems to relieve my feelings of being down.
16. I've been taking some steroids to help build up my body for the past 2 years.
17. I take the steroids in cycles (2 months on, 2 months off).
18. During the football season, I don't take steroids because we get tested.
19. I have had trouble maintaining an erection for the past 3 months.
20. I have anxiety about sex and being able to perform.
21. I am allergic to penicillin.

PHYSICAL CHECKLIST

1. Performed an ophthalmoscopic examination in both eyes
2. Listened to the lungs posteriorly (side to side 4 levels)
3. Examined the heart
4. Examined thyroid anteriorly and posteriorly
5. Palpated the abdomen *AFTER* auscultation in all 4 quadrants
6. Inspected nasal septum.

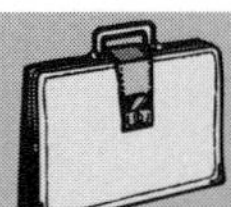

SP's Communication and Interpersonal Skills (CIS) Checklist

1. Knocked before entering
2. Opened interview by introducing self
3. Addressed patient using last name with introduction (e.g., Mr. Milano)
4. Appearance (e.g., clean and neat)
5. Allowed patient to express reason for seeking medical attention
6. Made comfortable eye contact
7. Did *not* use leading/biased questions (e.g., "You don't have…" or "You're not…")
8. Asked questions individually
9. Did *not* use the "Why" question
10. Concentrated and focused on patient's needs
11. Maintained comfortable and appropriate distance
12. Gave patient time to think and answer without interrupting
13. Used proper draping during physical exam
14. Did physical examination in an orderly manner
15. Summarized patient's condition (or asked patient to summarize)
16. Discussed diagnostic tests and/or next step in treatment in lay terms
17. Asked whether patient had other questions/concerns
18. Provided patient education/suggestions where appropriate
19. Did *not* give false assurances
20. Showed empathy

123 SP's Spoken English Proficiency (SEP) Rating Scale

	Poor	Fair	Good	Very Good	Excellent
1. Ability of *patient* to understand *candidate*	1	2	3	4	5
2. Ability of *candidate* to understand *patient*	1	2	3	4	5
3. Candidate is articulate	1	2	3	4	5
4. Words are pronounced correctly	1	2	3	4	5
5. Range of vocabulary and sentence structure	1	2	3	4	5
6. Stress, rhythm, and intonation	1	2	3	4	5
7. Grammar	1	2	3	4	5
8. Repair strategies	1	2	3	4	5

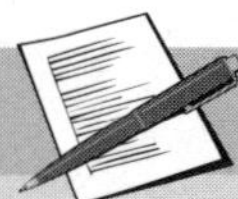

Example of a Satisfactory Patient Note (PN)

HISTORY—Include any significant pertinent positives and negatives

Mr. Jacques Milano is a 17-year-old high school senior who has been in good health for most of his life. He presents today for medical evaluation at the insistence of his football coach.

Ten months ago, his father died suddenly, after which he noticed that he has been "feeling down." He had been very close to his father. Now he has had great difficulty concentrating; his grades are slipping; and he has early morning awakening. To try to feel better, he started snorting cocaine about 5 months ago.

He's a high school athlete playing football and hopes to get sports scholarship to college, but he is now worried about getting one because of his bad grades. He also admits to steroid use for the past 2 years on a 2-month-on, 2-month-off cycle. He also drinks 3–4 cans of beer on the weekend. He denies other recreational drug use.

He lives at home with his mother, younger sister, and younger brother. He has had five girlfriends, and he has slept with four of them. He uses condoms. There is no history of any STD. Recently he has noted that he is having difficulty with erections and is worried about that.

He is allergic to penicillin; he gets a rash.

PHYSICAL EXAMINATION—Include any significant pertinent positives and negatives

Physical examination reveals an extremely well-developed, well-nourished, 17-year-old, appearing his stated age, with acne on his face and back. Vital signs are normal except for a diastolic BP of 85. Nasal septum is intact. Ophthalmoscopic examination reveals normal discs and vasculature. Thyroid exam is within WNL. Examination of the chest is clear to auscultation and percussion. Cardiac exam reveals the PMI to be in the 5th ICS-MCL; S_1 and S_2 are WNL; there are no murmurs, rubs, or gallops heard. Examination of the abdomen is normal.

DIFFERENTIAL DIAGNOSIS

In order of likelihood, write no more than five (5) differential diagnoses

1. Substance abuse (cocaine, steroids)
2. Depression
3. __________
4. __________
5. __________

DIAGNOSTIC WORKUP

Immediate plans, write no more than five (5) diagnostic studies

1. Male genital exam
2. Blood toxicology screen
3. T_3, TSH, CBC, serum testosterone
4. __________
5. __________

CASE 26—Ms. Erica Warren

Ms. Erica Warren, a 49-year-old woman, presents to clinic complaining of recurrent cough.

VITAL SIGNS

Temperature: 99.2° F	**Pulse:** 85 regular
Blood Pressure: 130/70	**Respiratory Rate:** 14 regular

EXAMINEE'S TASKS

In the next 15 minutes, you are to:

1. Take a focused history
2. Do a focused physical examination
3. Discuss your initial clinical impressions and workup plans with the patient
4. Write the Patient Note after leaving the room

Examinee's Data Gathering (DG) Checklists

HISTORY CHECKLIST

1. ______________________
2. ______________________
3. ______________________
4. ______________________
5. ______________________
6. ______________________
7. ______________________
8. ______________________
9. ______________________
10. ______________________
11. ______________________
12. ______________________
13. ______________________
14. ______________________
15. ______________________
16. ______________________
17. ______________________
18. ______________________
19. ______________________
20. ______________________

PHYSICAL EXAMINATION CHECKLIST

1. ______________________
2. ______________________
3. ______________________
4. ______________________
5. ______________________
6. ______________________

7. ______________________________
8. ______________________________

Total DG Score _____ *Passing Score for DG is 20 points (70%)*

Examinee's Communication and Interpersonal Skills (CIS) Checklist

1. ______________________________
2. ______________________________
3. ______________________________
4. ______________________________
5. ______________________________
6. ______________________________
7. ______________________________
8. ______________________________
9. ______________________________
10. ______________________________
11. ______________________________
12. ______________________________
13. ______________________________
14. ______________________________
15. ______________________________
16. ______________________________
17. ______________________________
18. ______________________________
19. ______________________________
20. ______________________________

Total CIS Score _____ *Passing Score for CIS is 14 points (70%)*

123 Examinee's Spoken English Proficiency (SEP) Rating Scale

	Poor	Fair	Good	Very Good	Excellent
1. Ability of *patient* to understand *candidate*	1	2	3	4	5
2. Ability of *candidate* to understand *patient*	1	2	3	4	5
3. Candidate is articulate	1	2	3	4	5
4. Words are pronounced correctly	1	2	3	4	5
5. Range of vocabulary and sentence structure	1	2	3	4	5
6. Stress, rhythm, and intonation	1	2	3	4	5
7. Grammar	1	2	3	4	5
8. Repair strategies	1	2	3	4	5

Total SEP Score ______ *Passing Score for SEP is 28 points (70%)*

Examinee's Patient Note (PN)

HISTORY—Include any significant pertinent positives and negatives

PHYSICAL EXAMINATION—Include any significant pertinent positives and negatives

DIFFERENTIAL DIAGNOSIS

In order of likelihood, write no more than five (5) differential diagnoses

1.
2.
3.
4.
5.

DIAGNOSTIC WORKUP

Immediate plans, write no more than five (5) diagnostic studies

1.
2.
3.
4.
5.

Even if you are pretty sure of a diagnosis, be aware that it is generally inappropriate to give the patient a definitive diagnosis during the examination. One reason is that you are dressed and the patient is not, leaving them vulnerable and perhaps not as able to think as clearly as they will when they are dressed in their usual attire. After you have ordered and received the results of tests, you will see the patient in your office to discuss the results and provide them with the diagnosis in a more appropriate setting.

Background Information for Standardized Patient

PATIENT BEHAVIOR

Coughs throughout the interview

AFFECT

Upset; concerned; looking to the doctor for real help

PROVOCATIVE QUESTION(S) AND PLAUSIBLE ANSWER(S)

"I've got this terrible cough. Do you think this is cancer?"

"It's still too early to know. We need to perform a physical examination and do some laboratory tests. As soon as I have all the results, I will discuss them with you."

ADDITIONAL NOTES

Have a red-stained tissue paper in the garbage

CHIEF COMPLAINT

"I've got a bad cough."

HISTORY OF PRESENT ILLNESS

Erica Warren is a 49-year-old woman who comes to clinic today for evaluation of a recurrent cough. About 5 months ago, she started coughing. At first, it was mostly in the afternoon, but now it's all day and even awakens her from sleep. She is also becoming increasingly short of breath. About 2 months ago, she started bringing up thick sputum. It's yellow in color and doesn't smell bad. For the past month, she noticed that sometimes the sputum was blood-tinged. Yesterday, she coughed up a clot of blood, became real scared, and decided to come in for evaluation. She has tried some over-the-counter cough medications, but they don't seem to work. She thinks that she may have a fever, but she doesn't have a thermometer. She has no chills, but on occasion, she has had night sweats. She has lost about 9 pounds in the past 3 months; she doesn't seem to have an appetite. She also doesn't have the energy she had before the cough began.

PAST MEDICAL HISTORY

She has a history of converting to a positive PPD about 8 years ago when she was working in the hospital. She was given INH to take for 1 year, which she did.

MEDICATIONS

Albuterol inhaler

ALLERGIES

None

SOCIAL HISTORY

She is a retired nurse's aide, and she has worked in several hospitals. She was a heavy smoker and smoked about 2 packs per day for about 25 years. Since her cough began, she has cut back to about 5 cigarettes a day. She doesn't drink or use recreational drugs.

FAMILY HISTORY

Her mother, age 73, has diabetes. Her father died of heart failure and lung disease at age 68. He was a big smoker. She has two sisters, ages 51 and 47. They are in good health.

SEXUAL HISTORY

She has been married for 22 years and has a 19-year-old son. She is sexually active with only her husband, but because of the cough, she has not had sexual relations for about 2 months.

REVIEW OF SYSTEMS

Noncontributory

SP's Data Gathering (DG) Checklists

HISTORY CHECKLIST

1. I've got a bad cough.
2. I've had this cough for about 5 months.
3. At first, it was mostly in the afternoon, but now it's all day and even awakens me from sleep.
4. I am becoming increasingly short of breath.
5. About 2 months ago, I started bringing up thick sputum.
6. The sputum is yellow in color and doesn't smell bad.
7. I have noticed that for the past month my sputum has been blood-tinged.
8. Yesterday, I coughed up a clot of blood.
9. I tried some over-the-counter cough medications, but they don't seem to work.
10. I think that I might have a fever, but I don't have a thermometer.
11. I don't have any chills, but on occasion, I have had night sweats.
12. I've lost about 9 pounds in the past 3 months.
13. I just don't seem to have an appetite.
14. I had a positive PPD about 8 years ago when I was working in the hospital.
15. I was given INH to take for 1 year.
16. I take my albuterol inhaler when I need it for shortness of breath.
17. I have no allergies.
18. I am a retired nurse's aide and have worked in several hospitals.
19. I was a heavy smoker and smoked about 2 packs per day for about 25 years.
20. Since my cough began, I have cut back to about 5 cigarettes a day.

PHYSICAL CHECKLIST

1. Evaluated lymph nodes of head, neck, and axilla
2. Evaluated heart by auscultation
3. Evaluated anterior lung fields (4 levels) by palpation (tactile fremitus)
4. Evaluated anterior lung fields (4 levels) by percussion
5. Evaluated anterior lung fields (4 levels) by auscultation
6. Evaluated posterior lung fields (4 levels) by palpation (tactile fremitus)
7. Evaluated posterior lung fields (4 levels) by percussion
8. Evaluated posterior lung fields (4 levels) by auscultation

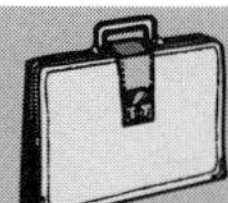

SP's Communication and Interpersonal Skills (CIS) Checklist

1. Knocked before entering
2. Opened interview by introducing self
3. Addressed patient using last name with introduction (e.g., Ms. Warren)
4. Appearance (e.g., clean and neat)
5. Allowed patient to express reason for seeking medical attention
6. Made comfortable eye contact
7. Did *not* use leading/biased questions (e.g., "You don't have..." or "You're not...")
8. Asked questions individually
9. Did *not* use the "Why" question
10. Concentrated and focused on patient's needs
11. Maintained comfortable and appropriate distance
12. Gave patient time to think and answer without interrupting
13. Used proper draping during physical exam
14. Did physical examination in an orderly manner
15. Summarized patient's condition (or asked patient to summarize)
16. Discussed diagnostic tests and/or next step in treatment in lay terms
17. Asked whether patient had other questions/concerns
18. Provided patient education/suggestions where appropriate
19. Did *not* give false assurances
20. Showed empathy

123 SP's Spoken English Proficiency (SEP) Rating Scale

	Poor	Fair	Good	Very Good	Excellent
1. Ability of *patient* to understand *candidate*	1	2	3	4	5
2. Ability of *candidate* to understand *patient*	1	2	3	4	5
3. Candidate is articulate	1	2	3	4	5
4. Words are pronounced correctly	1	2	3	4	5
5. Range of vocabulary and sentence structure	1	2	3	4	5
6. Stress, rhythm, and intonation	1	2	3	4	5
7. Grammar	1	2	3	4	5
8. Repair strategies	1	2	3	4	5

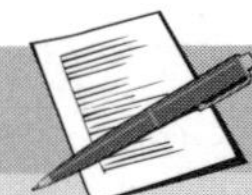

Example of a Satisfactory Patient Note (PN)

HISTORY—Include any significant pertinent positives and negatives

Ms. Erica Warren is a 49-year-old woman who presents to the clinic with the complaint of "I've got a bad cough."

HISTORY OF PRESENT ILLNESS

- Cough started about 5 months ago; at first, it was mostly in the afternoon, but now it's all day and awakens patient from sleep
- Becoming increasingly short of breath
- About 2 months ago, thick, yellow-colored sputum which doesn't smell bad started to be produced
- Recently within the past month, sputum has been blood-tinged; yesterday patient coughed up a clot of blood
- Tried over-the-counter cough medications, but without relief
- Patient doesn't have a thermometer but thinks she may have a fever
- (+) occasional night sweats
- (−) chills
- (+) 9-pound weight loss in past 3 months; no appetite
- (+) positive PPD about 8 years ago when working as a nurse's aide in the hospital; given INH to take for 1 year
- Takes albuterol inhaler for shortness of breath

PAST MEDICAL HISTORY

- Medications
  Albuterol inhaler as needed
- (−) allergies

SOCIAL HISTORY

- Retired nurse's aide and worked in several hospitals
- Married, one son, age 22
- Smokes—2 packs per day for 25 years; now down to 5 cigarettes per day since cough began
- (−) recreational drug use

FAMILY HISTORY

- Mother—73 years old, diabetes
- Father died—heart failure and lung disease, age 68
- 2 Sisters—ages 51 and 47, A&W

REVIEW OF SYSTEMS

- Noncontributory

PHYSICAL EXAMINATION—Include any significant pertinent positives and negatives

GENERAL

- Physical examination reveals a well-developed, slightly obese, 49-year-old woman appearing her stated age and complaining of recurrent cough

VITAL SIGNS

- BP 130/70
- 99.2° F
- Otherwise WNL

LYMPH NODES

- (–) posterior cervical, occipital, tonsillar, anterior auricular, posterior auricular, maxillary, submental, or axillary adenopathy

CHEST

- Clear to P&A—no evidence of consolidation or effusions; no crackles or rubs heard

CARDIAC

- PMI 5th ICS-MCL
- S_1S_2 WNL
- (–) murmurs, gallops, or rubs appreciated

DIFFERENTIAL DIAGNOSIS

In order of likelihood, write no more than five (5) differential diagnoses

1. Lung cancer
2. Tuberculosis
3. COPD
4. Pneumonia
5. Bronchiectasis

DIAGNOSTIC WORKUP

Immediate plans, write no more than five (5) diagnostic studies

1. Chest x-ray
2. CBC, blood cultures
3. Pulmonary function tests
4. Sputum—Gram stain and culture, AFB smear and mycobacterial culture, cytology
5. CT of chest

CASE 27—Ms. Denise Butterfield

Ms. Denise Butterfield, a 25-year-old woman, presents to clinic complaining of right knee pain.

VITAL SIGNS

Temperature: 99.9° F	**Pulse:** 80 regular
Blood Pressure: 130/70	**Respiratory Rate:** 14 regular

EXAMINEE'S TASKS

In the next 15 minutes, you are to:

1. Take a focused history
2. Do a focused physical examination
3. Discuss your initial clinical impressions and workup plans with the patient
4. Write the Patient Note after leaving the room

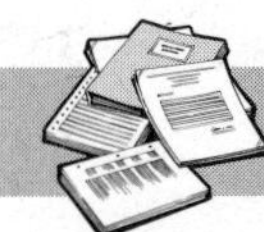

Examinee's Data Gathering (DG) Checklists

HISTORY CHECKLIST

1. ______
2. ______
3. ______
4. ______
5. ______
6. ______
7. ______
8. ______
9. ______
10. ______
11. ______
12. ______
13. ______
14. ______
15. ______
16. ______
17. ______
18. ______
19. ______
20. ______
21. ______
22. ______

PHYSICAL EXAMINATION CHECKLIST

1. ______
2. ______
3. ______
4. ______
5. ______
6. ______

Total DG Score ______ *Passing Score for DG is 20 points (70%)*

Examinee's Communication and Interpersonal Skills (CIS) Checklist

1. __________
2. __________
3. __________
4. __________
5. __________
6. __________
7. __________
8. __________
9. __________
10. __________
11. __________
12. __________
13. __________
14. __________
15. __________
16. __________
17. __________
18. __________
19. __________
20. __________

Total CIS Score ______ *Passing Score for CIS is 14 points (70%)*

123 Examinee's Spoken English Proficiency (SEP) Rating Scale

	Poor	Fair	Good	Very Good	Excellent
1. Ability of *patient* to understand *candidate*	1	2	3	4	5
2. Ability of *candidate* to understand *patient*	1	2	3	4	5
3. Candidate is articulate	1	2	3	4	5
4. Words are pronounced correctly	1	2	3	4	5
5. Range of vocabulary and sentence structure	1	2	3	4	5
6. Stress, rhythm, and intonation	1	2	3	4	5
7. Grammar	1	2	3	4	5
8. Repair strategies	1	2	3	4	5

Total SEP Score ______ *Passing Score for SEP is 28 points (70%)*

Examinee's Patient Note (PN)

HISTORY—Include any significant pertinent positives and negatives

PHYSICAL EXAMINATION—Include any significant pertinent positives and negatives

DIFFERENTIAL DIAGNOSIS

In order of likelihood, write no more than five (5) differential diagnoses

1.
2.
3.
4.
5.

DIAGNOSTIC WORKUP

Immediate plans, write no more than five (5) diagnostic studies

1.
2.
3.
4.
5.

When a patient presents with pain, remember to be particularly careful on the physical exam in that area. Examine the other extremity first!

Background Information for Standardized Patient

PATIENT BEHAVIOR

Jittery, doesn't like doctors, and wants to get out of the exam room as quickly as possible.

AFFECT

Anxious; distrustful of the interview

PROVOCATIVE QUESTION(S) AND PLAUSIBLE ANSWER(S)

"What the hell is wrong with me? Just give me something for the pain, and let me the hell outta here!"

"Let me find out a little more information about the problem and then we'll do some tests. Then I'll be better able to answer your question."

ADDITIONAL NOTES

Do not allow candidate to fully extend or flex your right knee
Paint right knee red to appear inflamed

CHIEF COMPLAINT

"Terrible right knee pain for the past 3 days"

HISTORY OF PRESENT ILLNESS

Denise Butterfield is a 25-year-old woman who complains of right knee pain for the past 3 days. She awakened 3 days ago and could hardly get out of bed because of the severe, sharp pain in her right knee. It was especially bad walking down the stairs from her bedroom. She noticed that it felt hot and red. She took some Tylenol with codeine, and it felt better. It doesn't hurt too much if she doesn't walk. The pain is worse in the morning and gradually gets a little better as the day goes on. She describes the pain as about a 7 out of 10. She took her temperature yesterday, and it was 100.1° F. She has no chills.

She's never had anything like this before, but she did injure her right knee about 3 years ago playing soccer. She was hospitalized for 7 days and given something called vancomycin. She then took some medicines for about 2 weeks after she went home from the hospital.

She has no history of pain in other joints. She has noticed that her fingers and toes get a little blue when exposed to the cold. She has no history of tick bites or rashes. She has no history of seizures, weakness, or numbness.

PAST MEDICAL HISTORY

Noncontributory

MEDICATIONS

None

ALLERGIES

None

SOCIAL HISTORY

She has been an intravenous drug user for 8 years. She has used heroin, shrooms, X, LSD, and sometimes free-based coke. She uses about four $10 bags of heroin twice a day. She supports her habit by sleeping with whomever can get her high. She wasn't sleeping with men so much for the money as for the fix. She would rather get the drugs than the money to buy the drugs. She has tried detox, but it didn't work. She has never overdosed. She smokes 2 ppd × 9 years.

FAMILY HISTORY

She doesn't speak to her parents so she doesn't know much about them. She thinks they are alive. She has an older sister and brother but doesn't speak to them either.

SEXUAL HISTORY

She has sexual relations only with men. She has had multiple partners, and now has three contacts. She had gonorrhea once when she was 21 years old. She had a miscarriage, which occurred in the fifth month of her pregnancy, when she was 19. She is unmarried. She uses condoms most of the time. Her last menstrual period was last week.

REVIEW OF SYSTEMS

She has had frequent oral ulcers, most recently 2 weeks ago.

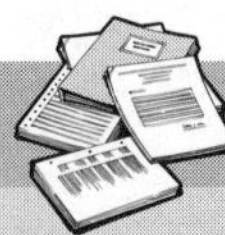

SP's Data Gathering (DG) Checklists

HISTORY CHECKLIST

1. I have this terrible right knee pain.
2. I woke up 3 days ago and could hardly get out of bed because of the severe, sharp pain in my right knee.
3. It was especially bad walking down the stairs from my bedroom.
4. The knee was hot and red.
5. I took some Tylenol with codeine, and it feels better.
6. It doesn't hurt too much if I don't walk.
7. The pain is worse in the morning and gradually gets a little better as the day goes on.
8. The pain is about a 7 out of 10.
9. I took my temperature yesterday; it was 100.1° F.
10. I have no chills.
11. I injured my right knee about 3 years ago playing soccer.
12. I was hospitalized for 7 days and given something called vancomycin.
13. I have no pain in my other joints.
14. I've noticed that my fingers and toes get a little blue when they are exposed to the cold.
15. I have no history of tick bites or rashes.
16. I have no history of seizures.
17. I have no weakness.
18. I have no numbness.
19. I have been an intravenous drug user for 8 years.
20. I've had multiple male sexual partners; now I have three contacts.
20. I had a miscarriage when I was 19; it occurred in the fifth month of my pregnancy.
21. I had gonorrhea when I was 21.
22. I have no allergies.

PHYSICAL CHECKLIST

1. Examined mouth for ulcerations
2. Evaluated heart by auscultation
3. Evaluated knees for tenderness
4. Evaluated knees for range of motion
5. Evaluated other joints (e.g., shoulders, elbows, wrists) for tenderness
6. Evaluated other joints (e.g., shoulders, elbows, wrists) for range of motion

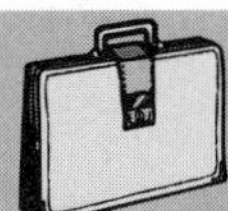

SP's Communication and Interpersonal Skills (CIS) Checklist

1. Knocked before entering
2. Opened interview by introducing self
3. Addressed patient using last name with introduction (e.g., Ms. Butterfield)
4. Appearance (e.g., clean and neat)
5. Allowed patient to express reason for seeking medical attention
6. Made comfortable eye contact
7. Did *not* use leading/biased questions (e.g., "You don't have…" or "You're not…")
8. Asked questions individually
9. Did *not* use the "Why" question
10. Concentrated and focused on patient's needs
11. Maintained comfortable and appropriate distance
12. Gave patient time to think and answer without interrupting
13. Used proper draping during physical exam
14. Did physical examination in an orderly manner
15. Summarized patient's condition (or asked patient to summarize)
16. Discussed diagnostic tests and/or next step in treatment in lay terms
17. Asked whether patient had other questions/concerns
18. Provided patient education/suggestions where appropriate
19. Did *not* give false assurances
20. Showed empathy

123 SP's Spoken English Proficiency (SEP) Rating Scale

	Poor	Fair	Good	Very Good	Excellent
1. Ability of *patient* to understand *candidate*	1	2	3	4	5
2. Ability of *candidate* to understand *patient*	1	2	3	4	5
3. Candidate is articulate	1	2	3	4	5
4. Words are pronounced correctly	1	2	3	4	5
5. Range of vocabulary and sentence structure	1	2	3	4	5
6. Stress, rhythm, and intonation	1	2	3	4	5
7. Grammar	1	2	3	4	5
8. Repair strategies	1	2	3	4	5

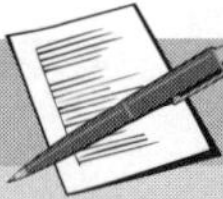

Example of a Satisfactory Patient Note (PN)

HISTORY—Include any significant pertinent positives and negatives

Ms. Denise Butterfield is a 25-year-old intravenous drug user who presents to clinic with the chief complaint of "terrible right knee pain for the past 3 days."

HISTORY OF PRESENT ILLNESS

- Severe, sharp right knee pain for past 3 days; knee described as hot and red
- Pain provoked by walking down the stairs
- Pain slightly improved with Tylenol with codeine or when knee is not bent
- Pain worse in the morning and gradually gets better as the day progresses
- Pain described as a 7 out of 10.
- (+) fever 100.1° F; (–) chills
- (+) injury right knee 3 years ago; hospitalized for 7 days and given vancomycin
- (–) pain in other joints
- (+) H/O Raynaud's
- (–) tick bites or rashes
- (–) seizures, weakness, numbness

PAST MEDICAL HISTORY

- (+) frequent oral ulcers, most recently 2 weeks ago
- (–) current medications
- (–) allergies

SOCIAL HISTORY

- (+) intravenous drug user for 8 years (heroin, shrooms, X, LSD, and sometimes free-based coke)
- Single, H/O multiple male sexual partners; now with three contacts
- Condom use "most of the time"
- (+) miscarriage in fifth month of pregnancy—age 19
- Smokes—2 ppd × 9 years
- (+) H/O gonorrhea, age 21

FAMILY HISTORY

- Mother—alive
- Father—alive
- Sister and brother

PHYSICAL EXAMINATION—Include any significant pertinent positives and negatives

GENERAL

- Physical examination reveals a well-developed, thin, 25-year-old woman appearing her stated age, holding her right knee and complaining of severe pain.

VITAL SIGNS

- BP 130/90
- 99.9° F
- Otherwise WNL

HEAD, EARS, EYES, NOSE, AND THROAT

- Mouth (–) ulceration

CHEST

- Clear to P&A

CARDIAC

- PMI 5th ICS-MCL
- S_1S_2 WNL
- (–) murmurs, gallops, rubs

EXTREMITIES

- Right knee—erythematous, edematous, and warm with limited range of motion; pain elicited on flexion and extension
- Left knee—WNL
- Shoulders, elbows, wrists—without evidence of inflammation; normal ranges of motion
- (+) track marks right and left forearms

DIFFERENTIAL DIAGNOSIS

In order of likelihood, write no more than five (5) differential diagnoses

1. Septic arthritis (gonococcal or nongonococcal)
2. Trauma (chondromalacia)
3. Rheumatologic disease (SLE or rheumatoid arthritis)
4. Lyme disease
5. Crystalline disease (gout or pseudogout)

DIAGNOSTIC WORKUP

Immediate plans, write no more than five (5) diagnostic studies

1. Knee arthrocentesis & synovial fluid analysis
2. CBC, ANA, anti-dsDNA, uric acid, Lyme antibody titer, RF, blood cultures
3. X-ray of knee
4. Pelvic exam & cervical cultures
5. ______________________________

CASE 28—Ms. Kathy Arden

Ms. Kathy Arden, a 41-year-old woman, presents to clinic complaining of palpitations.

VITAL SIGNS

Temperature: 98.6° F	**Pulse:** 70 regular
Blood Pressure: 130/70	**Respiratory Rate:** 12 regular

EXAMINEE'S TASKS

In the next 15 minutes, you are to:

1. Take a focused history
2. Do a focused physical examination
3. Discuss your initial clinical impressions and workup plans with the patient
4. Write the Patient Note after leaving the room

Examinee's Data Gathering (DG) Checklists

HISTORY CHECKLIST

1. ______
2. ______
3. ______
4. ______
5. ______
6. ______
7. ______
8. ______
9. ______
10. ______
11. ______
12. ______
13. ______
14. ______
15. ______
16. ______
17. ______
18. ______
19. ______
20. ______
21. ______
22. ______

PHYSICAL EXAMINATION CHECKLIST

1. ______
2. ______
3. ______
4. ______
5. ______

Total DG Score ______ *Passing Score for DG is 19 points (70%)*

Examinee's Communication and Interpersonal Skills (CIS) Checklist

1. ______
2. ______
3. ______
4. ______
5. ______
6. ______
7. ______
8. ______
9. ______
10. ______
11. ______
12. ______
13. ______
14. ______
15. ______
16. ______
17. ______
18. ______
19. ______
20. ______

Total CIS Score ______ *Passing Score for CIS is 14 points (70%)*

123 Examinee's Spoken English Proficiency (SEP) Rating Scale

	Poor	Fair	Good	Very Good	Excellent
1. Ability of *patient* to understand *candidate*	1	2	3	4	5
2. Ability of *candidate* to understand *patient*	1	2	3	4	5
3. Candidate is articulate	1	2	3	4	5
4. Words are pronounced correctly	1	2	3	4	5
5. Range of vocabulary and sentence structure	1	2	3	4	5
6. Stress, rhythm, and intonation	1	2	3	4	5
7. Grammar	1	2	3	4	5
8. Repair strategies	1	2	3	4	5

Total SEP Score ______ *Passing Score for SEP is 28 points (70%)*

Examinee's Patient Note (PN)

HISTORY—Include any significant pertinent positives and negatives

PHYSICAL EXAMINATION—Include any significant pertinent positives and negatives

DIFFERENTIAL DIAGNOSIS

In order of likelihood, write no more than five (5) differential diagnoses

1.
2.
3.
4.
5.

DIAGNOSTIC WORKUP

Immediate plans, write no more than five (5) diagnostic studies

1.
2.
3.
4.
5.

When you are dealing with a patient who appears not to trust doctors, it is advisable to show empathy, i.e., say an empathetic statement, as early in the interview as you can.

Background Information for Standardized Patient

PATIENT BEHAVIOR

Biting fingernails; tapping her foot; fiddling with her hair; speaking very quickly

AFFECT

Jittery; anxious; appears as if she can't wait to get out of the room; appears as if she doesn't like or trust the doctor

PROVOCATIVE QUESTION(S) AND PLAUSIBLE ANSWER(S)

"Look, can you help me? Not one of these doctors I've seen has been able to tell me what the hell is wrong with me!!"

"It's a good thing you came in. It must be very scary. We will absolutely do our best to help you to get to the bottom of why this is happening to you."

CHIEF COMPLAINT

"My heart is beating so fast. I'm so scared."

HISTORY OF PRESENT ILLNESS

Kathy Arden is a 41-year-old woman who comes to clinic for evaluation of palpitations (fluttering of heart beat) that awakened her last night from sleep. The palpitations lasted for about 20 minutes. She tried to gag herself and go to the bathroom and strain, but it didn't help. She just sat down and tried to do some relaxation exercises. She's been having palpitations since she was about 15 years old. She gets them about every 3–4 months. She has been seen by several doctors over the years. She was told a few years ago that she had a "bizarre ECG," but since then her ECGs have been pretty normal. She had several Holter monitors, but they showed nothing. One of the doctors advised her to take some medications, but she refused. He told her to do the gagging and straining maneuvers when she gets the palpitations. The episode last night was the worst one yet. She does not drink caffeinated beverages or eat chocolate.

She does not have a history of chest pain, lightheadedness, or shortness of breath associated with the palpitations.

PAST MEDICAL HISTORY

She has no history of heart or thyroid disease, but she was told as a child that she had a heart murmur.

MEDICATIONS

None

ALLERGIES
Cats

SOCIAL HISTORY
She is employed as a secretary in a luggage factory. She enjoys alcohol and drinks about 3–4 glasses of wine nightly. She also has been using cocaine whenever she can since she was about 18 years old. She last used cocaine about 3 days ago.

FAMILY HISTORY
Her mother, age 74, had breast cancer 5 years ago but is doing fine now. Her father, age 73, has had chronic lymphatic leukemia for 9 years and seems to be doing well. She is the youngest of five siblings—two brothers and three sisters—all alive and well.

SEXUAL HISTORY
She has never been married. She has been living with a man, with whom she is sexually active, for the past 4 years. She has no children.

REVIEW OF SYSTEMS
Noncontributory

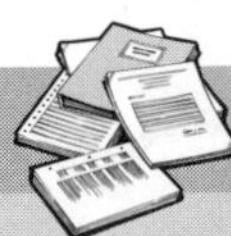

SP's Data Gathering (DG) Checklists

HISTORY CHECKLIST

1. My heart was beating so fast. I am so scared.
2. The palpitations awakened me from sleep last night.
3. They lasted for about 20 minutes.
4. I tried to gag myself and go to the bathroom and strain, but it didn't help.
5. I sat down and tried to do some relaxation exercises.
6. I've been having palpitations since I was about 15 years old.
7. I get them about every 3–4 months.
8. I was told a few years ago that I had a "bizarre ECG," but since then my ECGs have been pretty normal.
9. I had several Holter monitors, but they showed nothing.
10. One of my doctors advised me to take some medications, but I refused.
11. I was told to do the gagging and straining whenever I get the palpitations.
12. I do not have chest pain.
13. I do not have lightheadedness.
14. I do not have shortness of breath.
15. I was never told that I have thyroid disease.
16. I was told that I had a heart murmur as a child.
17. I do not take any medications.
18. I am allergic to cats.
19. I enjoy alcohol and drink about 3–4 glasses of wine nightly.
20. I do not drink caffeinated beverages or eat chocolate.
21. I have been using cocaine whenever I can since I was about 18 years old.
22. I last used cocaine about 3 days ago.

PHYSICAL CHECKLIST

1. Took blood pressure
2. Evaluated hair quality and texture
3. Evaluated thyroid by palpation, anteriorly and posteriorly
4. Evaluated the PMI
5. Evaluated the heart by auscultation (4 positions)

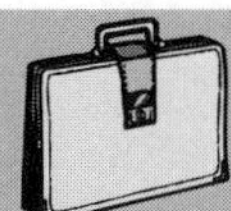

SP's Communication and Interpersonal Skills (CIS) Checklist

1. Knocked before entering
2. Opened interview by introducing self
3. Addressed patient using last name with introduction (e.g., Ms. Arden)
4. Appearance (e.g., clean and neat)
5. Allowed patient to express reason for seeking medical attention
6. Made comfortable eye contact
7. Did *not* use leading/biased questions (e.g., "You don't have..." or "You're not...")
8. Asked questions individually
9. Did *not* use the "Why" question
10. Concentrated and focused on patient's needs
11. Maintained comfortable and appropriate distance
12. Gave patient time to think and answer without interrupting
13. Used proper draping during physical exam
14. Did physical examination in an orderly manner
15. Summarized patient's condition (or asked patient to summarize)
16. Discussed diagnostic tests and/or next step in treatment in lay terms
17. Asked whether patient had other questions/concerns
18. Provided patient education/suggestions where appropriate
19. Did *not* give false assurances
20. Showed empathy

123 SP's Spoken English Proficiency (SEP) Rating Scale

	Poor	Fair	Good	Very Good	Excellent
1. Ability of *patient* to understand *candidate*	1	2	3	4	5
2. Ability of *candidate* to understand *patient*	1	2	3	4	5
3. Candidate is articulate	1	2	3	4	5
4. Words are pronounced correctly	1	2	3	4	5
5. Range of vocabulary and sentence structure	1	2	3	4	5
6. Stress, rhythm, and intonation	1	2	3	4	5
7. Grammar	1	2	3	4	5
8. Repair strategies	1	2	3	4	5

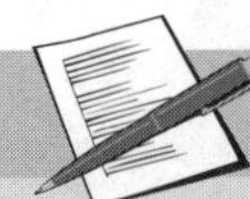

Example of a Satisfactory Patient Note (PN)

HISTORY—Include any significant pertinent positives and negatives

Ms. Kathy Arden is a 41-year-old woman who presents to clinic with the chief complaint of "My heart was beating so fast. I am so scared."

HISTORY OF PRESENT ILLNESS

- Palpitations awakened patient from sleep last night; lasted about 20 minutes; gagging and straining didn't help
- Has had palpitations since age 15 years old; occur about every 3–4 months
- Told a few years ago that she had a "bizarre ECG," but since then ECGs are said to be normal; (–) Holter monitoring
- (–) chest pain, lightheadedness, shortness of breath, thyroid disease
- (+) heart murmur as a child

PAST MEDICAL HISTORY

- (–) medications
- (+) allergies—cat

SOCIAL HISTORY

- Secretary in a luggage factory
- (+) alcohol 3–4 glasses of wine nightly
- (+) cocaine "whenever she can" since she was about 18 years old
- Last cocaine use about 3 days ago
- (–) caffeine

FAMILY HISTORY

- Mother—74 years old, breast cancer, age 69
- Father—73 years old, CLL × 9 years
- Patient is youngest of 5 siblings—all A&W

SEXUAL HISTORY

- Never married
- Living with a man for the past 4 years; no children

PHYSICAL EXAMINATION—Include any significant pertinent positives and negatives

GENERAL

- Physical examination reveals a well-developed, anxious, thin, 41-year-old woman appearing her stated age and complaining of palpitations.

VITAL SIGNS

- BP 130/70
- Otherwise WNL

HEAD, EARS, EYES, NOSE, AND THROAT

- Hair—firmly attached; normal texture
- Thyroid (–) masses, bruits, enlargement

CARDIAC

- PMI 5th ICS-MCL
- S_1S_2 WNL
- GII/VII late systolic murmur
- (–) gallops or rubs

DIFFERENTIAL DIAGNOSIS

In order of likelihood, write no more than five (5) differential diagnoses

1. Mitral valve prolapse
2. Hyperthyroidism
3. Supraventricular re-entrant tachycardia (e.g., WPW)
4. Drug-induced arrhythmia (e.g., cocaine, alcohol)
5. Panic disorder

DIAGNOSTIC WORKUP

Immediate plans, write no more than five (5) diagnostic studies

1. ECG
2. Holter monitor
3. CBC, TSH, free T_4, toxicology screen
4. Echocardiogram
5. ______________________________

CASE 29—Ms. Janice Gardner

Ms. Janice Gardner, a 25-year-old woman, presents to the emergency room complaining of abdominal pain.

VITAL SIGNS

Temperature: 99.3° F	**Pulse:** 95 regular
Blood Pressure: 120/65	**Respiratory Rate:** 14 regular

EXAMINEE'S TASKS

In the next 15 minutes, you are to:

1. Take a focused history
2. Do a focused physical examination
3. Discuss your initial clinical impressions and workup plans with the patient
4. Write the Patient Note after leaving the room

Examinee's Data Gathering (DG) Checklists

HISTORY CHECKLIST

1. ______
2. ______
3. ______
4. ______
5. ______
6. ______
7. ______
8. ______
9. ______
10. ______
11. ______
12. ______
13. ______
14. ______
15. ______
16. ______
17. ______
18. ______
19. ______

PHYSICAL EXAMINATION CHECKLIST

1. ______
2. ______
3. ______
4. ______
5. ______
6. ______

7. ______________________________
8. ______________________________

Total DG Score ______ *Passing Score for DG is 19 points (70%)*

Examinee's Communication and Interpersonal Skills (CIS) Checklist

1. ______________________________
2. ______________________________
3. ______________________________
4. ______________________________
5. ______________________________
6. ______________________________
7. ______________________________
8. ______________________________
9. ______________________________
10. ______________________________
11. ______________________________
12. ______________________________
13. ______________________________
14. ______________________________
15. ______________________________
16. ______________________________
17. ______________________________
18. ______________________________
19. ______________________________
20. ______________________________

Total CIS Score ______ *Passing Score for CIS is 14 points (70%)*

123 Examinee's Spoken English Proficiency (SEP) Rating Scale

	Poor	Fair	Good	Very Good	Excellent
1. Ability of *patient* to understand *candidate*	1	2	3	4	5
2. Ability of *candidate* to understand *patient*	1	2	3	4	5
3. Candidate is articulate	1	2	3	4	5
4. Words are pronounced correctly	1	2	3	4	5
5. Range of vocabulary and sentence structure	1	2	3	4	5
6. Stress, rhythm, and intonation	1	2	3	4	5
7. Grammar	1	2	3	4	5
8. Repair strategies	1	2	3	4	5

Total SEP Score ______ *Passing Score for SEP is 28 points (70%)*

Examinee's Patient Note (PN)

HISTORY—Include any significant pertinent positives and negatives

PHYSICAL EXAMINATION— Include any significant pertinent positives and negatives

DIFFERENTIAL DIAGNOSIS

In order of likelihood, write no more than five (5) differential diagnoses

1.
2.
3.
4.
5.

DIAGNOSTIC WORKUP

Immediate plans, write no more than five (5) diagnostic studies

1.
2.
3.
4.
5.

Remember that although you do want to pinpoint what is medically wrong with the patient, you are treating the entire person. One of your primary jobs, especially on the Step 2-CS exam, is to calm the patient down as much as possible, and reassure them that they have come to the right place and that you will do everything possible to help them.

Background Information for Standardized Patient

PATIENT BEHAVIOR

Shallow breathing; moving around as little as possible; lying still on stretcher holding right lower area of abdomen; grimacing in pain; uncomfortable discussing her sexual history but will do so if done in a gentle manner.

AFFECT

Scared; in extreme pain

CHIEF COMPLAINT

"Severe right lower belly pain"

HISTORY OF PRESENT ILLNESS

Janice Gardner is a 25-year-old woman who comes to the emergency room for evaluation of right lower abdominal pain. She describes the acute onset of severe right lower abdominal pain about 3 hours ago. It is very sharp in quality. Nothing seems to make it better. Moving makes the pain worse. It is about a 9 out of 10 in severity. She does not feel it in any other part of her body. She also has nausea and vomited twice. The vomit was yellow in color; there was no blood. She does not have diarrhea or constipation. She has no pain on urination or blood in her urine. She did notice this morning some brown vaginal spotting.

She is monogamous with her husband of 2 years. They have been trying to have children for the past year. She does not use any form of contraception. Her husband does not use condoms. Her last menstrual period was 7 weeks ago, which is not unusual for her as her periods are very irregular. Her last Pap smear was 8 months ago.

PAST MEDICAL HISTORY

She had a history of a heart murmur as a child.

MEDICATIONS

None

ALLERGIES

None

SOCIAL HISTORY

She is a third year medical student. She does not smoke, drink alcohol, or use other recreational drugs.

FAMILY HISTORY

Her mother, age 52, is alive and well. Her father, age 56, has Crohn's disease but is doing well. She has one brother, age 21, who is a senior in college. He is fine.

SEXUAL HISTORY

See History of Present Illness. Before her marriage, she had two other boyfriends with whom she was sexually active. She started having periods at age 12. They have always been irregular. They last for 4–5 days. She uses 4–5 tampons on the first 1–2 days. She has never had any sexually transmitted disease.

REVIEW OF SYSTEMS

Noncontributory

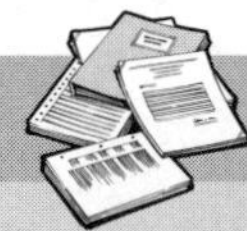

SP's Data Gathering (DG) Checklists

HISTORY CHECKLIST

1. I've got severe right lower belly pain.
2. It started about 3 hours ago.
3. It is very sharp in quality.
4. Nothing seems to make it better.
5. Moving makes the pain worse.
6. It is about a 9 out of 10 in severity.
7. I do not feel it in any other part of my body.
8. I am nauseated and vomited twice.
9. The vomit was yellow in color.
10. There was no blood.
11. I do not have diarrhea or constipation.
12. I do not have pain on urination.
13. I do not have blood in my urine.
14. I did notice this morning some brown vaginal spotting.
15. I am monogamous with my husband of 2 years.
16. We have been trying to have children for the past year.
17. We do not use any form of contraception.
18. My last menstrual period was 7 weeks ago, which is not unusual for me as my periods are very irregular.
19. My last Pap smear was 8 months ago.

PHYSICAL CHECKLIST

1. Took blood pressure
2. Evaluated bowel sounds
3. Performed light palpation of the abdomen in all 4 quadrants *after* auscultation
4. Performed deep palpation of the abdomen in all 4 quadrants
5. Elicited for rebound abdominal tenderness
6. Percussed abdomen in all 4 quadrants
7. Evaluated for psoas, Rovsing's, and/or obturator signs
8. Evaluated for CVA tenderness

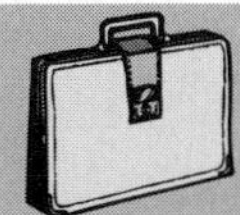

SP's Communication and Interpersonal Skills (CIS) Checklist

1. Knocked before entering
2. Opened interview by introducing self
3. Addressed patient using last name with introduction (e.g., Ms. Gardner)
4. Appearance (e.g., clean and neat)
5. Allowed patient to express reason for seeking medical attention
6. Made comfortable eye contact
7. Did *not* use leading/biased questions (e.g., "You don't have..." or "You're not...")
8. Asked questions individually
9. Did *not* use the "Why" question
10. Concentrated and focused on patient's needs
11. Maintained comfortable and appropriate distance
12. Gave patient time to think and answer without interrupting
13. Used proper draping during physical exam
14. Did physical examination in an orderly manner
15. Summarized patient's condition (or asked patient to summarize)
16. Discussed diagnostic tests and/or next step in treatment in lay terms
17. Asked whether patient had other questions/concerns
18. Provided patient education/suggestions where appropriate
19. Did *not* give false assurances
20. Showed empathy

123 SP's Spoken English Proficiency (SEP) Rating Scale

	Poor	Fair	Good	Very Good	Excellent
1. Ability of *patient* to understand *candidate*	1	2	3	4	5
2. Ability of *candidate* to understand *patient*	1	2	3	4	5
3. Candidate is articulate	1	2	3	4	5
4. Words are pronounced correctly	1	2	3	4	5
5. Range of vocabulary and sentence structure	1	2	3	4	5
6. Stress, rhythm, and intonation	1	2	3	4	5
7. Grammar	1	2	3	4	5
8. Repair strategies	1	2	3	4	5

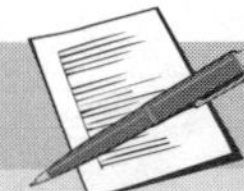

Example of a Satisfactory Patient Note (PN)

HISTORY—Include any significant pertinent positives and negatives

Ms. Janice Gardner is a 25-year-old sexually active woman who presents to the ER with the chief complaint of "severe right lower belly pain."

HISTORY OF PRESENT ILLNESS

- Pain, very sharp in quality, started about 3 hours ago
- Nothing seems to make it better; moving makes the pain worse
- It is about a 9 out of 10 in severity
- (–) radiation
- (+) nausea
- (+) vomited twice; vomit yellow in color, (–) blood
- (+) brown vaginal spotting this AM
- (–) diarrhea or constipation
- (–) dysuria, hematuria
- LMP 7 weeks ago, which is not unusual as periods are very irregular
- Last Pap smear was 8 months ago

PAST MEDICAL HISTORY

- (+) heart murmur as child
- (–) current medications
- (–) allergies

SOCIAL HISTORY

- Medical student
- Married × 2 years, no children
- Trying to have children × 2 years
- No contraception
- (–) smoking
- (–) recreational drug use
- (–) STDs

FAMILY HISTORY

- Mother—52 years old, A&W
- Father—56 years old—Crohn's disease
- Brother—age 21, A&W

PHYSICAL EXAMINATION—Include any significant pertinent positives and negatives

GENERAL

- Physical examination reveals a well-developed, 25-year-old woman appearing her stated age, complaining of right lower quadrant abdominal pain, and holding her abdomen

VITAL SIGNS

- BP 130/70
- 99.3° F
- Otherwise WNL

ABDOMEN

- (+) BS
- (+) tenderness RLQ
- (–) masses
- (–) rebound tenderness
- (+) psoas (right)
- (–) Rovsing's, obturator signs
- (–) CVAT

DIFFERENTIAL DIAGNOSIS

In order of likelihood, write no more than five (5) differential diagnoses

1. Ectopic pregnancy
2. Ovarian torsion
3. Ruptured ovarian cyst
4. Pelvic inflammatory disease
5. Appendicitis

DIAGNOSTIC WORKUP

Immediate plans, write no more than five (5) diagnostic studies

1. Pelvic and rectal exams
2. Ultrasound of abdomen & pelvis
3. Urine hCG
4. CBC, amylase, BUN, creatinine
5. CT of abdomen & pelvis

CASE 30—Mr. Leo Mandel

Mr. Leo Mandel, a 30-year-old man, presents to clinic complaining of diarrhea and abdominal pain.

VITAL SIGNS

Temperature: 98.9° F	**Pulse:** 85 regular
Blood Pressure: 125/80	**Respiratory Rate:** 12 regular

EXAMINEE'S TASKS

In the next 15 minutes, you are to:

1. Take a focused history
2. Do a focused physical examination
3. Discuss your initial clinical impressions and workup plans with the patient
4. Write the Patient Note after leaving the room

Examinee's Data Gathering (DG) Checklists

HISTORY CHECKLIST

1. ___
2. ___
3. ___
4. ___
5. ___
6. ___
7. ___
8. ___
9. ___
10. ___
11. ___
12. ___
13. ___
14. ___
15. ___
16. ___
17. ___
18. ___
19. ___
20. ___
21. ___
22. ___
23. ___

PHYSICAL EXAMINATION CHECKLIST

1. ___
2. ___
3. ___
4. ___
5. ___

6. ______________________________
7. ______________________________

Total DG Score ______ *Passing Score for DG is 21 points (70%)*

Examinee's Communication and Interpersonal Skills (CIS) Checklist

1. ______________________________
2. ______________________________
3. ______________________________
4. ______________________________
5. ______________________________
6. ______________________________
7. ______________________________
8. ______________________________
9. ______________________________
10. ______________________________
11. ______________________________
12. ______________________________
13. ______________________________
14. ______________________________
15. ______________________________
16. ______________________________
17. ______________________________
18. ______________________________
19. ______________________________
20. ______________________________

Total CIS Score ______ *Passing Score for CIS is 14 points (70%)*

123 Examinee's Spoken English Proficiency (SEP) Rating Scale

	Poor	Fair	Good	Very Good	Excellent
1. Ability of *patient* to understand *candidate*	1	2	3	4	5
2. Ability of *candidate* to understand *patient*	1	2	3	4	5
3. Candidate is articulate	1	2	3	4	5
4. Words are pronounced correctly	1	2	3	4	5
5. Range of vocabulary and sentence structure	1	2	3	4	5
6. Stress, rhythm, and intonation	1	2	3	4	5
7. Grammar	1	2	3	4	5
8. Repair strategies	1	2	3	4	5

Total SEP Score ______ *Passing Score for SEP is 28 points (70%)*

Examinee's Patient Note (PN)

HISTORY—Include any significant pertinent positives and negatives

PHYSICAL EXAMINATION— Include any significant pertinent positives and negatives

DIFFERENTIAL DIAGNOSIS

In order of likelihood, write no more than five (5) differential diagnoses

1.
2.
3.
4.
5.

DIAGNOSTIC WORKUP

Immediate plans, write no more than five (5) diagnostic studies

1.
2.
3.
4.
5.

Background Information for Standardized Patient

PATIENT BEHAVIOR
Lying on stretcher; moving very little

AFFECT
Frightened

PROVOCATIVE QUESTION(S) AND PLAUSIBLE ANSWER(S)
"Do you think I have cancer?"

"It's highly unlikely, but let's get a few tests done first, and then we'll have a better idea of what's going on."

ADDITIONAL NOTES
Holding lower abdomen

Blood in the toilet bowl always produces anxiety, especially for a man who has never seen it before. Of course, any woman would also be anxious if she saw blood which came from her GI tract. Show empathy by stating, "That must be very scary."

CHIEF COMPLAINT
"Diarrhea and abdominal pain for the past 2 months"

HISTORY OF PRESENT ILLNESS
Leo Mandel is a 30-year-old man who has been having diarrhea and abdominal pain for the past 2 months. He came for evaluation today because he noticed that there was some red blood mixed in with the stool, and he got very scared.

He first noted having abdominal pain with watery diarrhea, however, about 1 year ago when he was traveling with a friend in Latin America. He took some Pepto-Bismol and Imodium, which was given to him by his friend, for the pain and diarrhea. The pain persisted on and off for about 2 weeks and then disappeared.

The symptoms returned about 2 months ago, except that the diarrhea now is no longer watery; however, the stool is very loose. The pain is crampy in nature and is relieved with elimination (*i.e., defecation*). He says that he feels the pain all over his abdomen, but it is most centered around his belly button. He describes the pain as about a 6 out of 10. He also has a bloating sensation in his abdomen. He does not have any nausea, vomiting, or weight loss. He saw a local MD about 3 weeks ago who gave him some antibiotic that seemed to make things worse, so he stopped taking it after 5 days. The symptoms still persist. He has had about 10 bowel movements a day for the past week. There is now some mucus mixed in with the stool.

PAST MEDICAL HISTORY
He had a benign tumor removed from his tongue when he was 16 years old. No other surgery.

MEDICATIONS

None

ALLERGIES

None

SOCIAL HISTORY

He is single and lives with his girlfriend of 7 months. He uses marijuana about one or twice a month. He doesn't use any other recreational drugs.

FAMILY HISTORY

His mother is 50 years old and is in good heath. His father is 52 and has a "weak stomach."

SEXUAL HISTORY

He is monogamous with his girlfriend. He has had about six girlfriends and has slept with five of them. He uses condoms.

REVIEW OF SYSTEMS

When he was 19 years old, he had iritis in both his eyes. He was treated with topical steroids and dilators. He also has a history of low back pain which he thinks he got after too much bowling. The pain is intermittent and started when he was about 23 years old.

SP's Data Gathering (DG) Checklists

HISTORY CHECKLIST

1. I've been having diarrhea and abdominal pain for the past 2 months.
2. I came today because I noticed that there was some red blood mixed in with the stool.
3. I first had abdominal pain with watery diarrhea about 1 year ago.
4. I was traveling with a friend in Latin America.
5. I took some Pepto-Bismol and Imodium for the pain and diarrhea.
6. The pain persisted on and off for about 2 weeks and then disappeared.
7. The diarrhea now is very loose, not watery, stools.
8. The pain is crampy.
9. The pain is relieved with elimination.
10. I feel the pain all over my abdomen, but it is most centered around my belly button.
11. The pain is about a 6 out of 10.
12. I also feel a bloating sensation in my abdomen.
13. I do not have any nausea.
14. I have not been vomiting.
15. I have not had any weight loss.
16. A local physician gave me an antibiotic, which made things worse.
17. I have had 10 bowel movements a day for the past week.
18. There is now some mucus mixed in with the stool.
19. I had iritis in both eyes when I was 19 years old.
20. I was treated with topical steroids and dilators.
21. I have had low back pain since I was about 23 years old.
22. I like to smoke pot once or twice a month.
22. I have no allergies.
23. My parents are alive and well; mom is 50 and dad is 52 and has a weak stomach.

PHYSICAL CHECKLIST

1. Inspected mouth for oral ulcers
2. Performed light palpation of the abdomen in all 4 quadrants *after* auscultation
3. Performed deep palpation of the abdomen in all 4 quadrants
4. Performed percussion of the abdomen
5. Evaluated liver size
6. Evaluated liver by palpation
7. Evaluated sacroiliac joints for tenderness

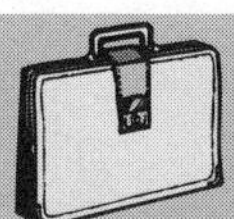

SP's Communication and Interpersonal Skills (CIS) Checklist

1. Knocked before entering
2. Opened interview by introducing self
3. Addressed patient using last name with introduction (e.g., Mr. Mandel)
4. Appearance (e.g., clean and neat)
5. Allowed patient to express reason for seeking medical attention
6. Made comfortable eye contact
7. Did *not* use leading/biased questions (e.g., "You don't have…" or "You're not…")
8. Asked questions individually
9. Did *not* use the "Why" question
10. Concentrated and focused on patient's needs
11. Maintained comfortable and appropriate distance
12. Gave patient time to think and answer without interrupting
13. Used proper draping during physical exam
14. Did physical examination in an orderly manner
15. Summarized patient's condition (or asked patient to summarize)
16. Discussed diagnostic tests and/or next step in treatment in lay terms
17. Asked whether patient had other questions/concerns
18. Provided patient education/suggestions where appropriate
19. Did *not* give false assurances
20. Showed empathy

123 SP's Spoken English Proficiency (SEP) Rating Scale

	Poor	Fair	Good	Very Good	Excellent
1. Ability of *patient* to understand *candidate*	1	2	3	4	5
2. Ability of *candidate* to understand *patient*	1	2	3	4	5
3. Candidate is articulate	1	2	3	4	5
4. Words are pronounced correctly	1	2	3	4	5
5. Range of vocabulary and sentence structure	1	2	3	4	5
6. Stress, rhythm, and intonation	1	2	3	4	5
7. Grammar	1	2	3	4	5
8. Repair strategies	1	2	3	4	5

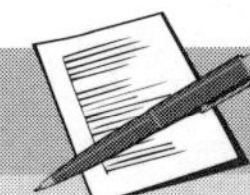

Example of a Satisfactory Patient Note (PN)

HISTORY—Include any significant pertinent positives and negatives

Mr. Leo Mandel is a 30-year-old who has come to clinic with the chief complaint of "diarrhea and abdominal pain."

HISTORY OF PRESENT ILLNESS

- Diarrhea & abdominal pain × 2 months
- Very loose, not watery, stool
- Physician gave antibiotic, which made things worse
- 10 bowel movements a day for the past week
- (+) blood in stool this AM
- (+) mucus
- (+) bloating sensation in his abdomen
- Pain is crampy; all over abdomen, but mostly centered around belly button
- Relieved with elimination
- 6 out of 10 in severity
- (–) nausea, vomiting, or weight loss

PAST MEDICAL HISTORY

- Abdominal pain with watery diarrhea about 1 year ago when traveling in Latin America
- Took some Pepto-Bismol and Imodium for the pain and diarrhea
- Pain persisted on and off for about 2 weeks and then disappeared
- H/O iritis in both his eyes, age 19, treated with topical steroids and dilators
- H/O low back pain since age 23
- No allergies

SOCIAL HISTORY

- Smokes pot 1–2 times a month

FAMILY HISTORY

- Mother—A&W—age 50
- Father—Alive—age 52—"weak stomach"

PHYSICAL EXAMINATION—Include any significant pertinent positives and negatives

GENERAL

- Well-developed, slightly thin, pale, 30-year-old man appearing his stated age, complaining of moderate abdominal pain and diarrhea

VITAL SIGNS

- WNL

HEAD, EARS, EYES, NOSE, AND THROAT

- (−) oral ulcers

ABDOMEN

- Slightly distended; (+) bowel sounds; mild tenderness throughout abdomen; tympany throughout abdomen; no masses present; liver span 10 cm in the midclavicular line; liver nontender

MUSCULOSKELETAL

- (−) sacroiliac tenderness

DIFFERENTIAL DIAGNOSIS

In order of likelihood, write no more than five (5) differential diagnoses

1. Inflammatory bowel disease
2. Irritable bowel disease
3. Pseudomembranous (C. *difficile*) colitis
4. Traveler's diarrhea
5. Celiac disease

DIAGNOSTIC WORKUP

Immediate plans, write no more than five (5) diagnostic studies

1. Rectal exam and stool for FOBT, stool for ova and parasites, *Clostridium difficile* toxin in stool
2. Abdominal x-ray
3. CBC, Na^+, K^+, Cl^-, TSH, AST, ALT, bilirubin
4. Colonoscopy
5. CT of abdomen

Appendix A

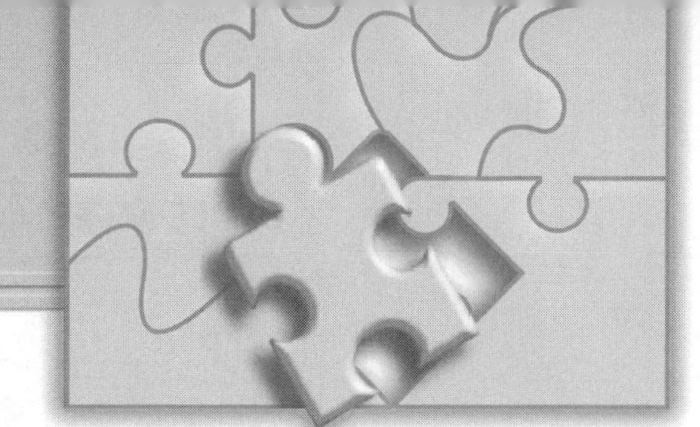

Acceptable Abbreviations

USMLE ACCEPTABLE ABBREVIATIONS FOR THE PATIENT NOTE

yo	year-old
m	male
f	female
b	black
w	white
L	left
R	right
hx	history
h/o	history of
c/o	complaining of
NL	normal limits
WNL	within normal limits
Ø	without or no
+	positive
–	negative
Abd	abdomen
ABG	arterial blood gas
AIDS	acquired immune deficiency syndrome
AP	anteroposterior
BUN	blood urea nitrogen
CABG	coronary artery bypass grafting
CBC	complete blood count
CCU	cardiac care unit
CHF	congestive heart failure
cig	cigarettes
COPD	chronic obstructive pulmonary disease
CPR	cardiopulmonary resuscitation
CT	computed tomography
CVA	cerebrovascular accident
CVP	central venous pressure
CXR	chest x-ray

USMLE ACCEPTABLE ABBREVIATIONS FOR THE PATIENT NOTE

DM	diabetes mellitus
DTR	deep tendon reflexes
ECG	electrocardiogram
ED	emergency department
EMT	emergency medical technician
ENT	ears, nose, and throat
EOM	extraocular muscles
ER	emergency room
ETOH	alcohol
Ext	extremities
FH	family history
GI	gastrointestinal
GU	genitourinary
HEENT	head, eyes, ears, nose, and throat
HIV	human immunodeficiency virus
HPI	history of present illness
HTN	hypertension
IM	intramuscularly
IV	intravenously
JVD	jugular venous distention
KUB	kidney, ureter, and bladder
LMP	last menstrual period
LP	lumbar puncture
MI	myocardial infarction
MRI	magnetic resonance imaging
MVA	motor vehicle accident
Neuro	neurologic
NIDDM	non–insulin-dependent diabetes mellitus
NKA	no known allergies
NKDA	no known drug allergy
NSR	normal sinus rhythm
PA	posteroanterior
PERRL	pupils equal, round, react to light (also known as PERRLA)
PMH	past medical history
po	orally
PT	prothrombin time
PTT	partial prothrombin time
RBC	red blood cells
ROS	review of systems
SH	social history
TIA	transient ischemic attack
U/A	urinalysis
URI	upper respiratory tract infection
WBC	white blood cells

Appendix B

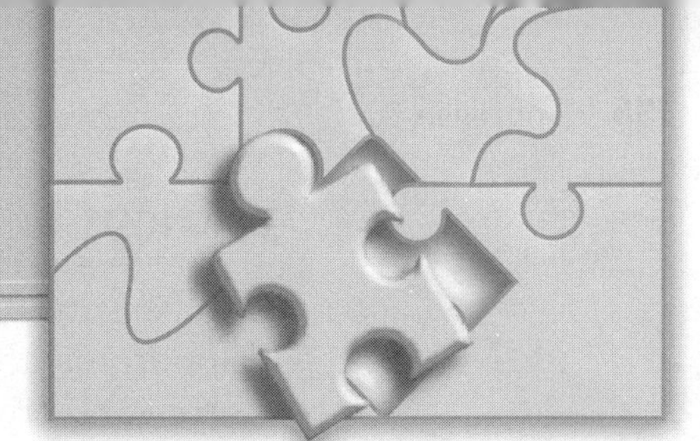

Possible Case Diagnoses

DIAGNOSIS	CASE(S)
Achalasia	12
Acoustic neuroma	11
AIDS	18
Alzheimer's disease	17
Anxiety disorder	24
Aortic dissection	22
Appendicitis	29
Arthritis, degenerative	3
Arthritis, rheumatoid	27
Arthritis, septic	27
Asbestosis	7
Asthma, viral-induced (child)	15
Atrophic endometrium	14
Benign positional vertigo	11
Benign prostatic hyperplasia	10
Berry aneurysm, ruptured	6
Brain tumor	1
Bronchiectasis	26
Cancer, cervical	14
Cancer, colorectal	19
Cancer, endometrial	14
Cancer, esophageal	12
Cancer, gastric	12
Cancer, hepatocellular	13
Cancer, lung	7, 26
Cancer, pancreatic	24
Cancer, prostate	10
Cancer, renal cell	10
Cardiac syncope	20
Carpal tunnel syndrome	4
Celiac disease	30

DIAGNOSIS	CASE(S)
Cholecystitis	2, 13
Chondromalacia	27
Chronic obstructive pulmonary disease	7, 16, 26
Congestive heart failure	16
Congestive heart failure (child)	15
Conversion disorder	5
Coronary artery disease	8, 22
Costochondritis	22
Cryptococcosis	18
Crystalline disease (gout, pseudogout)	27
Depression	1, 24, 25
Diabetes mellitus	5, 23
Diastolic cardiac dysfunction	16
Disc herniation, acute	3
Diverticulosis	19
Drug-induced arrhythmia (e.g., cocaine, alcohol)	28
Endometrial hyperplasia, drug-induced	14
Endometrial polyps	14
Erectile dysfunction, diabetes-related	9
Erectile dysfunction, drug-related	9
Erectile dysfunction, hypothyroidism-related	9
Erectile dysfunction, psychogenic	9
Esophageal stricture	12
Esophagitis, chronic	12
Familial benign tremor	20
Foreign-body aspiration (child)	15
Ganglion cyst	4
Gastritis	2
GERD	2, 22
Headache, migraine	1, 6
Headache, tension	1
Hematuria, exertional	10
Hemorrhoids	19
Hepatitis, acute alcoholic	13
Hepatitis, acute viral	13
Histoplasmosis	18
Hyperthyroidism	8, 23, 28
Hyperventilation	8
Hypothyroidism	17, 24
Inflammatory bowel disease	19, 30
Intracerebral hemorrhage, cocaine-induced	6
Intracranial tumor	17
Irritable bowel syndrome	30
Labyrinthitis	11
Lumbar muscular strain	3
Lyme disease	27

DIAGNOSIS	CASE(S)
Ménière's disease	11
Meningitis	6
Mesothelioma	7
Mitral valve prolapse	8, 28
Multi-infarct dementia	17
Multiple sclerosis	5
Occult malignancy	3, 23
Ovarian cyst, ruptured	29
Ovarian torsion	29
Pancreatitis	2, 13
Panic disorder	8, 28
Parkinson's disease	20
Pelvic inflammatory disease	29
Peptic ulcer disease	2
Pericarditis	22
Pleural fibrosis	7
Pneumonia	16, 26
Pneumonia (child)	15
Pneumonia, *Pneumocystis carinii*	18
Polycystic ovary syndrome	21
Posttraumatic stress syndrome	24
Pregnancy	21
Pregnancy, ectopic	29
Premature ovarian failure	21
Pseudomembranous colitis, *Clostridium difficile*	19, 30
Pulmonary emboli	16
Radiculopathy, cervical	4
Radiculopathy, ulnar	4
Spinal stenosis, lumbar	3
Stress-induced amenorrhea	21
Subarachnoid hemorrhage	6
Subdural hematoma	17
Substance abuse	25
Supraventricular re-entrant tachycardia (e.g., WPW)	28
Systemic lupus erythematosus	27
Temporal arteritis	1
Thyroid disease	20, 21
Transitional cell bladder tumor	10
Traveler's diarrhea	30
Tremor, drug-induced	20
Tuberculosis	18, 26
Tuberculosis (child)	15
Tumor, CNS	5
Vasculitis, CNS	5
Vestibular neuronitis	11

Index